Yoga for All
42 Essential Yoga Postures

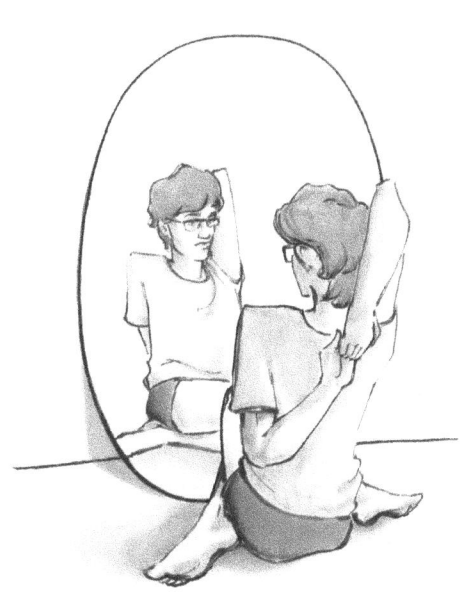

First edition 2021
Published by Alimentanima Books, Canberra, Australia

All images are the property of the artist Lisa Canogar and cannot be copied or stored without the written permission of the illustrator.

Copyright © Alimentanima Books 2021

ISBN: 978-0-6450732-1-8

Edited by: Nitya Dambiec
Illustrated by: Lisa Canogar

All rights reserved. No part of this publication may be reproduced, transmitted, or stored in a retrieval system in any form or by any means without the written permission of the publisher.

Yoga For All

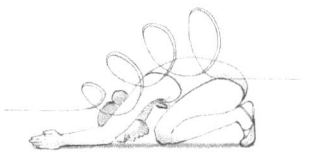

Illustrated by: Lisa Canogar
Edited by: Nitya Dambiec

Contents

Pg. 1- ABOUT THIS BOOK

1. *Yogásana* (Posture of the Yogi)
2. *Ardhakurmakásana* (Half-Tortoise Posture)
3. *Bhújauṇgásana* (Cobra Posture)
4. *Padahastásana* (Arm-and-Leg Posture)
5. *Karmásana* (Action Posture)
6. *Sarváuṇgásana* (Shoulder-Stand)
7. *Úrdhvapadmásana* (Upside-Down Lotus Posture)
8a. *Matsyamudrá* (Fish Posture 1)
8b. *Matsyásana* (Fish Posture 2)
9. *Naokásana* (Boat Posture)
10. *Utkata Paschimottánásana* (Back-Lifting Posture)
11. *Gomukhásana* (Cow's-Head Posture)
12. *Bhastrikásana* (Bellows Posture)
13. *Mayúrásana* (Peacock Posture)
14. *Matsyendrásana* (Posture of the Yogi Matsyendra)
15. *Cakrásana* (Wheel Posture)
16. *Garuḍásana* (Eagle Posture)
17. *Tuládaṅḍásana* (Balance Posture)
18. *Sahaja Utkatásana* (Simple Chair Posture)
19. *Jaṭila Utkatásana* (Difficult Chair Posture)
20. *Dvisamakoṅásana* (Double-Right-Angle Posture)
21. *Parvatásana* (Mountain Posture)
22. *Shivásana* (Posture of Shiva)

23. *Ardhashivásana* (Half-Shiva Posture)
24. *Tejásana* (Energy Posture)
25. *Jiṅánásana* (Knowledge Posture)
26. *Bhávásana* (Contemplation Posture)
27. *Shashàuṇgásana* (Hare Posture)
28. *Jánushiirásana* (Head-to-Knee Posture)
29. *Siddhásana* (Posture of Enlightenment)
30. *Padmásana* (Lotus Posture)
31. *Baddha Padmásana* (Tied-Lotus Posture)
32. *Vajrásana* (Lightening-Bolt Posture)
33. *Utkata Vajrásana* (Difficult Lightening-Bolt Posture)
34. *Shalabhásana* (Locust Posture)
35. *Uśtrásana* (Camel Posture)
36. *Kukkutásana* (Rooster Posture)
37. *Viirásana* (Hero's Posture)
38. *Kúrmakásana* (Tortoise Posture)
39. *Granthimuktásana* (Knot-Loosening Posture)
40. *Mańdukásana* (Frog Posture)
41. *Utkata Kúrmakásana* (Difficult Tortoise Posture)
42. *Shavásana* (Relaxation Posture)

Pg. 91- KAOSHIKII
Pg. 93- MODEL OF AN EFFECTIVE YOGA ROUTINE
Pg. 95- THE SATTVIC DIET

About this Book

This book, containing illustrations and instructions for forty-two essential yoga postures, or *'asanas,'* is designed to serve as a reference for students, practitioners and teachers alike. The postures are part of the Ananda Marga system of yoga and are designed to be incorporated into a regular, preferably daily, yoga practice. They can also be used in yoga classes. Each illustration is accompanied by instructions indicating how to correctly perform the posture, as well as a summary of its benefits. Variations and adjustments are not included, but anyone with a basic knowledge of yoga or stretching should easily be able to imagine and create variations on the original postures according to their or their student's physical capacity. The postures should be eased into step by step, without excessive force, and it should be remembered that it is more important to be comfortable than to perform them perfectly the first time.

In general, it recommended to practise yoga asanas under the guidance of a trained teacher. The Ananda Marga system of asanas is a personalised system, in which a specific combination of postures are selected for the practitioner according to their physical and emotional condition. Maximum benefit is received by the regular repetition of a few specially selected postures, rather than the mixing and changing of many different ones. The benefits given in this book are the most general ones, for commonly occurring physical as well as emotional problems. More specific benefits and therapeutic combinations are not included as these require the knowledge and experience of a teacher to be prescribed. The information given should, however, be enough to enable anyone to start a basic yoga practice even when personalised instruction is not available.

As well as being a useful reference and introduction to yoga asanas, this book also has another purpose. We hope that it expresses something of the spirit of yoga, as part of the collective knowledge of humanity, which should be available on a non-commercial basis for the benefit and well-being of all. Many thanks goes to the illustrator Lisa Canogar, who has made this book into a unique work of art reflecting the concept of 'unity in diversity', which was the vision of P. R. Sarkar, the spiritualist and humanist who founded this particular school of yoga, of which the physical postures are one small but important part. We hope that the images reflect this idea: of a yoga that is for people from all walks of life, ages, interests, genders and cultures, and that seeks, in addition to physical health and emotional balance, for a deepened understanding of our shared humanity.

Guidelines for a Successful Yoga Practice

Yoga asanas, in addition to maintaining the flexibility of the muscles and joints, are designed to aid in the balanced functioning of the lymphatic, nervous and endocrine systems, and in turn the health of the digestive and reproductive organs as well as the emotions. To receive all of these benefits, it is advisable to practice them according to a specific system: repeating the postures a certain numbers of times, holding them for a specified period of time, and with the proper breathing.

When practising asanas, many muscles that we normally are not aware of are stretched and strengthened. Special importance is given to the spinal column and the joints. The movements, which are at once gentle and firm, never forced, stimulate the circulation and flow of lymph. The lymphatic system, unlike the circulatory system, does not have its own pumping system, and depends on other bodily movements to circulate. The asanas, through repetition together with deep breathing, are designed especially to stimulate the movement of lymph throughout the entire body. The lymphatic system has an important role in maintaining the overall health of the organism, especially of the immune system, and in the prevention of infection and disease. After finishing your yoga routine, it is recommended to do a simple self-massage, which again stimulates the lymphatic system, as well as having a soothing effect on the nerves.

The repetitive movements of the postures, together with correct inhalation, exhalation and holding of the breath have a calming and strengthening effect on the nerves. The pressure placed at certain points of the body is considered to aid the proper functioning of the endocrine or glandular system and the hormonal secretions. This in turn affects the emotions, concentration, etc. and all the other bodily functions such as the digestion, circulation, urinary and reproductive functions. Yoga is a holistic system which speaks not of one or other isolated function, but rather of the interactions between different systems: the nervous system affects the glands, which affect the organs, which affect the lymphatic system, which in turn affects the glands, the emotions, and so on. The idea is to maintain a balanced functioning of the body as a whole, and as a result, support the proper functioning of the mind.

In order to receive the full benefits of an asana routine, in addition to following the repetition and breathing instructions, there are a few other tips that help. It is not recommended to practise asanas for at least two hours after eating. The best time to practise is in the morning before taking breakfast, or in the evening before taking dinner. Before practising, one should be calm and refreshed. If you have taken a shower before hand, that's perfect. Otherwise, there is a simple yogic system called 'half-bath', designed to refresh and relax the body and nerves, which can be done before starting your yoga routine. It only takes a minute, and can also be done before eating, sleeping, meditating, or whenever you feel rushed, tired or anxious. First, pour cool water from your knees to your feet, and then from the elbows to the hands. After this, breath in and place a handful of water in your mouth. Holding your breath, splash water into you open eyes at least twelve times. Spit out the water from your mouth and then wash your face and neck. With this, you are ready to start your yoga routine.

It is best to practice asanas indoors, away from the wind, sun or abrupt changes of temperature. Although yoga asanas are very useful in treating menstrual problems and other problems of the female reproductive system, it is not advisable to perform them during the menstruation period, due to the repetitive movements and resulting pressure placed on the glands and other fixed points of the body. During your period, other light stretches can be practised, without the repetition or specific breathing patterns, but it is better not to do the yoga postures in their original form. The postures which help to alleviate menstrual pain and other irregularities are cited, and practised the rest of the month, before and after menstruation, are very beneficial. The postures in this book are not suitable for pregnant mothers or during the weeks directly after childbirth. During these times other light stretches can be practised. For children, asanas can be done as stretching exercises, but the breathing, holding and repetition of the positions is not necessary.

For those who are new to yoga asanas and do not know where to begin, three basic postures have been recommended for women, and four for men. They have been selected to maintain the general health and flexibility of the body and reproductive system. These postures are quick to perform and can easily be incorporated into one's daily routine. They can be used as a base upon which other postures can then be added. In general, it is sufficient to perform four to six different postures in one sitting. The three basic postures recommended for women are numbers 1, 2 and 3; for men, numbers 6, 8a, 9 and 10.

On completing your yoga routine it is highly recommended to finish with a simple self massage and 2-10 minutes of relaxation. This helps the body to assimilate all the benefits of the asanas. The self-massage is done by first placing your hands over your eyes for a moment in order to relax them, and then passing them lightly over your face, neck, and entire body, paying special attention to the joints. You can give an extra massage to your feet. This is a massage of the skin, not the muscles, so there is no need to use pressure. After this, lie on you back in the relaxation posture (number 42), breathing deeply.

At the end of the book we have included instructions for a yogic dance called 'kaoshikii,' which can be practised at any time or be incorporated into your asana routine. It is designed to stretch the entire body, stimulate the lymphatic system and balance the nerves and glands. It is very beneficial for both men and women, but has special benefits for the female body. It can be practised even during pregnancy if desired, when adjusted to the physical condition of the mother. The dance can be repeated as many times and as slowly or quickly as desired. The name 'kaoshikii' means 'a dance to open up the layers of the mind.' As well as being beneficial to the physical health, it is designed to stimulate the nerves and glands in a way that, with regular and continued practice, also has positive psychological effects, helping to develop strength of mind and overcome anxiety, melancholy and fear.

Finally, you will find an index with some basic information about the yogic diet and food types that help to prepare the body and mind to receive maximum benefit from your yoga practice, as well as some additional tips. Good luck and enjoy your yogic adventure!

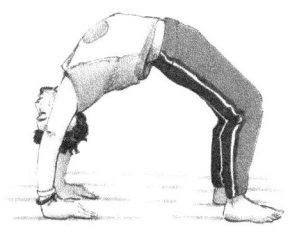

1. Yogásana
(Posture of the Yogi)

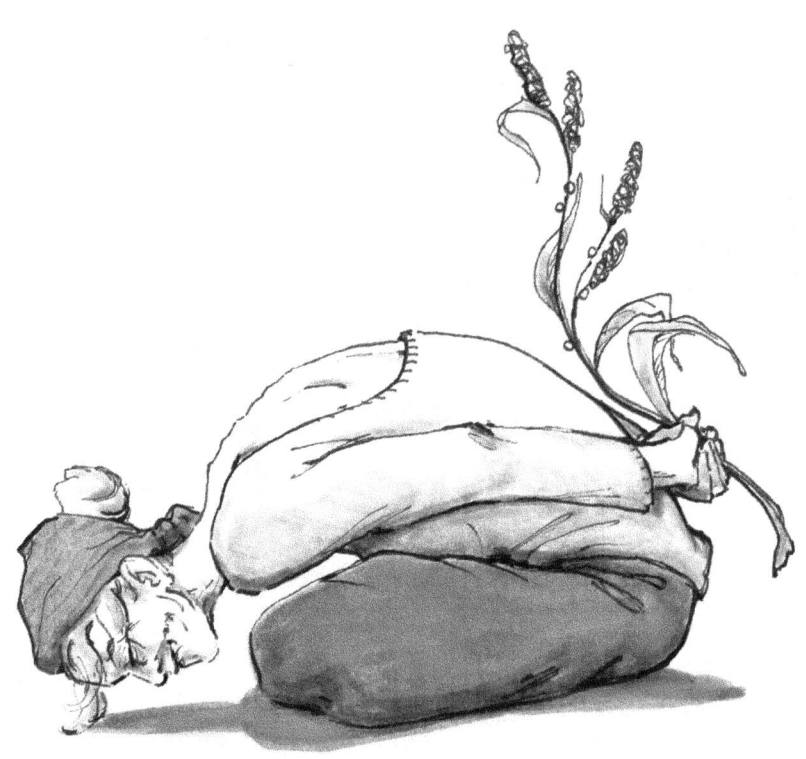

Instructions

1. Sit with your legs crossed. Hold your left wrist with your right hand.
2. Breathing out, bend forwards until your forehead and nose are touching the floor.
3. Hold this position for eight seconds, without breathing (breath exhaled).
4. Slowly sit up straight again. Breathe in as you raise your body. Repeat eight times.

- This is one of the three basic yoga postures recommended for women to help maintain all-round good health and the proper functioning of the female reproductive system. It is recommended for those suffering from menstrual cramps, irregular menstruation, etc. (Although especially useful for women, it is also very beneficial for men).
- Helps to develop good digestion and flexibility of the spine.

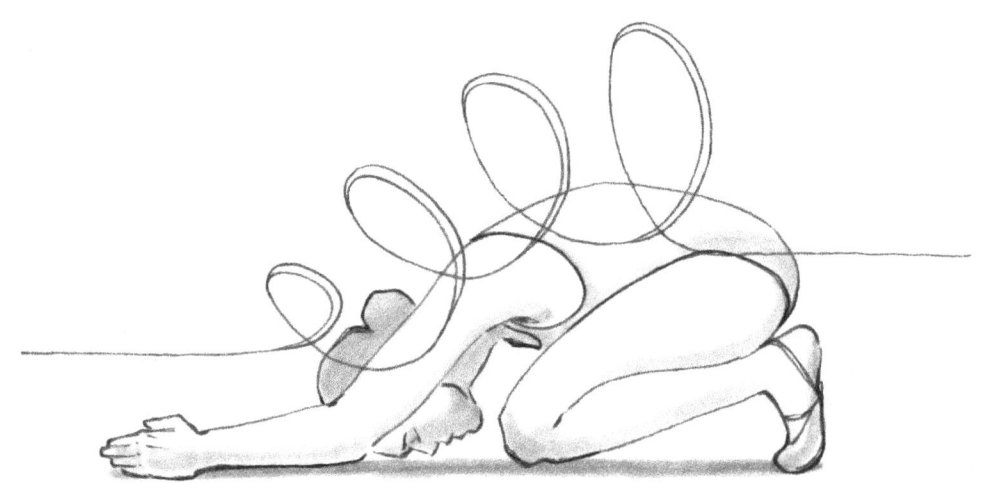

2. Ardhakurmakásana
(Half-Tortoise Posture)

Instructions

1. Kneel on the floor, with your toes facing forwards (inwards) and your buttocks resting on your heels.
2. Extend your arms upwards, bringing your palms together above your head. Keep your arms straight and always close to your ears.
3. Bend forwards, exhaling, until your nose and forehead touch the ground, keeping your buttocks always touching your heels. Your arms should be extended straight ahead and your palms should remain together.
4. Hold this position for eight seconds without breathing (breath exhaled).
5. Breathe in as you raise your body to return to the original position. Repeat eight times.

- This is one of the three basic yoga postures recommended for women to help maintain all-round good health and the proper functioning of the female reproductive system. It is recommended for those suffering from menstrual cramps, irregular menstruation, etc. (Although especially useful for women, it is also very beneficial for men).
- Helpful in treating loss of appetite, weakness of the stomach muscles and excessive accumulation of abdominal fat.
- Helps to develop good digestion and flexibility of the spine.

3. *Bhújauṋgásana* (Cobra Posture)

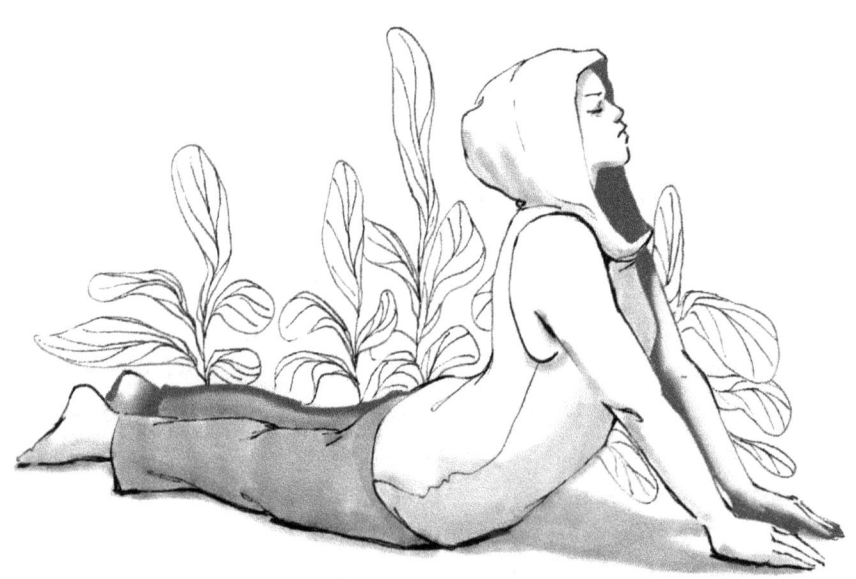

Instructions

1. Lie down on the floor, face to the ground, with your hands placed next to your shoulders.
2. Supporting your weight on your palms, inhale and raise your chest, directing your head slightly backwards as if looking towards the roof. Your navel should remain close to or touching the floor. Hold this position for eight seconds without breathing (breath inhaled).
3. Breathing out, relax your body and return to the original position, lying on the floor. Repeat eight times.

- This is one of the three basic yoga postures recommended for women to help maintain all-round good health and the proper functioning of the female reproductive system. It is recommended for those suffering from menstrual cramps, irregular menstruation, etc. (Although especially useful for women, it is also very beneficial for men).
- Helps to maintain the flexibility of the spinal cord and to strengthen the abdominal region.
- Helpful in treating digestive problems and maintaining a healthy digestive system.

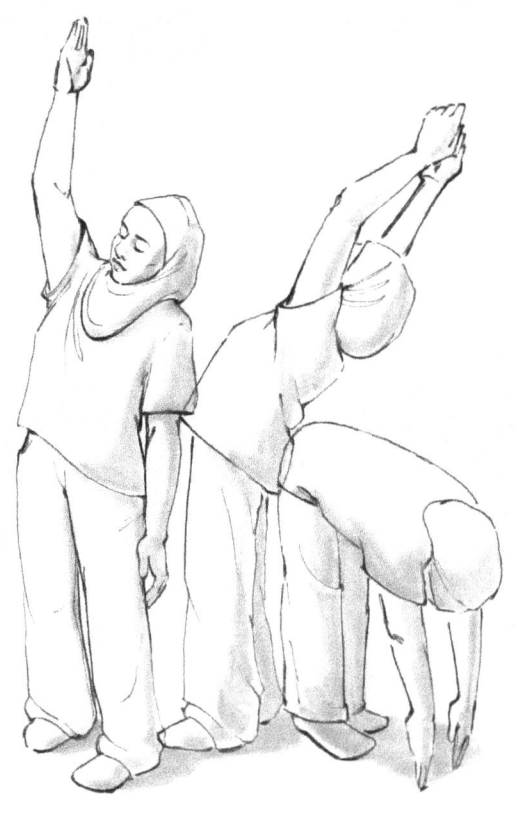

4. *Padahastásana* (Arm-and-Leg Posture)

Instructions

1. Stand with your feet apart at the same distance as your shoulders. Raise your arms, with your palms held open. Bend as far as possible to the right, breathing out. Maintain this position without breathing (breath exhaled) for eight seconds.
2. Raise your arms to the centre again, breathing in. Bend to the left, breathing out, and hold for eight seconds in the same way.
3. Raise your arms to the centre, breathing in. Breathe out, bend forwards, and hold your toes with your hands (without bending your knees). Maintain this position for eight seconds, without breathing (breath exhaled).
4. Breathe in, raise your arms to the centre, and then stretch backwards as far as possible. Maintain this position for eight seconds, without breathing (breath inhaled).
5. Breathe out, bending forwards to touch your big toes, and then immediately breathe in again and raise your arms upwards to the centre.
6. Repeat this process eight times.

- Helps to maintain all-round good health and flexibility. This posture can be easily practised by those who have difficulty doing other postures or who have reduced mobility.
- Helpful in treating menstrual problems (cramps, irregularity, etc.).
- Beneficial for those with weak health or who are recovering from illness.

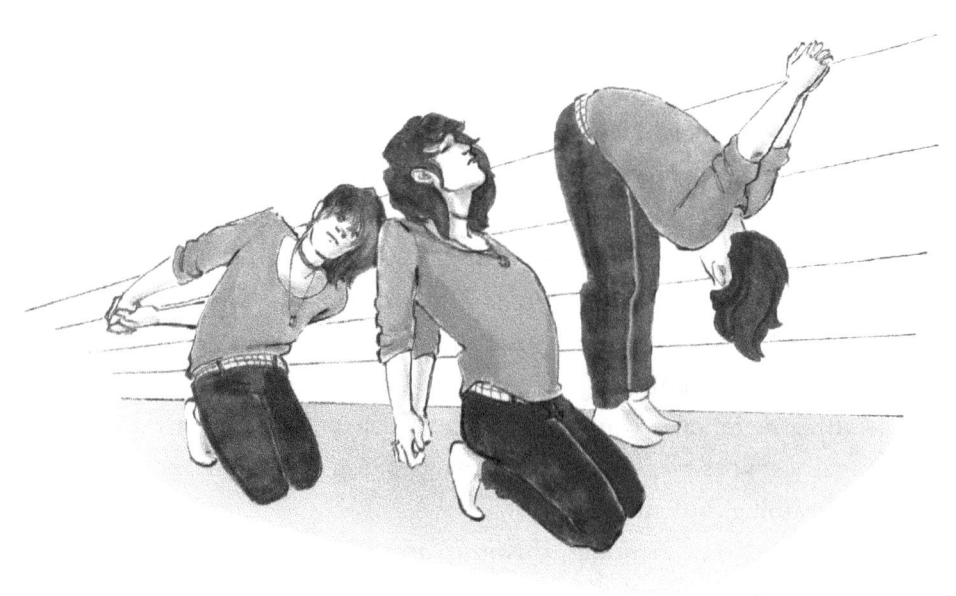

5. *Karmásana* (Action Posture)

This posture is made up of two parts. Complete the first part once, followed by the second part. Repeat this process four times.

Instructions

PART 1

1. Stand with your feet apart, at the same distance as your shoulders. Interlink your fingers behind your back.
2. Bend your body to the left (your arms will move to the right), breathing out. Hold this position for eight seconds without breathing (breath exhaled). Inhale and return to the centre.
3. Next, bend to the right, breathing out, and hold this position for eight seconds.
4. After this, bend forwards, breathing out and raising your arms upwards. Hold this position for eight seconds without breathing. Finally, stretch backwards, breathing in and holding the position for eight seconds.

PART 2

1. Repeat the same pattern as in the first part, but kneeling on the floor instead of standing, with your buttocks resting on your heels and toes facing inwards (forwards).
2. When bending forwards, your nose and forehead should touch the ground. You can raise your buttocks from your feet as your bend.
3. When bending backwards, your hands should touch the ground near your feet, helping to support the weight of your body.

- Helps to maintain over-all good health and flexibility of the entire body.
- This posture makes one active and energetic. It is helpful for people who suffer from physical weakness and fatigue.
- Useful for women suffering from menstrual cramps and other menstrual problems.

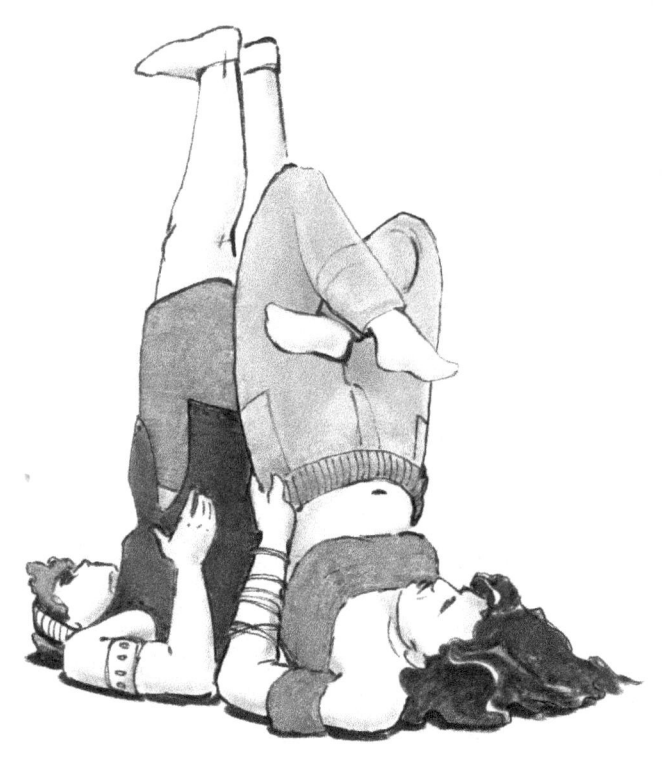

6. Sarváuṇgásana (Shoulder-Stand)
7. Úrdhvapadmásana (Upside-Down Lotus Posture)

Instructions

1. For *sarváuṇgásana,* lie on your back and gradually raise your legs and back until the weight of your body is supported by your shoulders. Your chin should be in contact with your chest. Support both sides of your back with your hands. Your feet should be held together and your eyes should look towards your toes.
2. For *úrdhvapadmásana,* place your right foot on your left thigh, and then your left foot on your right thigh, as in *padmásana* (lotus posture). Slowly lie down on your back, keeping your legs in this position. Then raise your body, proceeding as with *sarváuṇgásana.*
3. Practise three times, for a maximum of five minutes each time, breathing normally.
4. It is recommended to alternate this posture with *matsyamudrá* (fish posture), which should be practised for half the duration of *sarváuṇgásana/úrdhvapadmásana.* For example, do *sarváuṇgásana* for three minutes, followed by *matsyamudrá* for one and a half minutes.

- This is one of the four basic postures recommended for men, to maintain overall good health, mental balance and the proper functioning of the male reproductive system. (It is also very beneficial for women.)
- Helpful for those who have a weak immune system and often fall sick.
- Recommended for problems of the thyroid and parathyroid glands and metabolism.
- Helps to develop good concentration.

- *After the age of 60, if one suffers from high blood pressure, this posture should not be practised.*

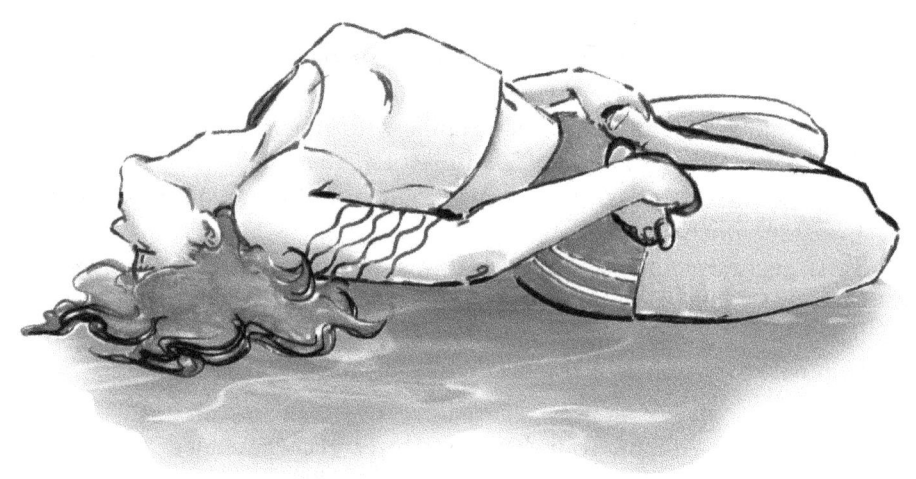

8a. Matsyamudrá **(Fish Posture 1)**

Instructions

1. Place your right foot on your left thigh, and then your left foot on your right thigh, as in *padmásana* (lotus posture). Rest the crown of your head on the floor, with your spine curved upwards. Hold your big toes with your hands.
2. Practise three times, breathing normally. It is recommended to alternate this posture with *sarváuṇgásana,* in which case it should be done for half the length of *sarváuṇgásana.* For example, do *sarváuṇgásana* for three minutes, followed by *matsyamudrá* for one and a half minutes. The maximum time of practice should be no more than two and a half minutes (preceded by *sarváuṇgásana* for five minutes).

- This is one of the four basic postures recommended for men, to maintain overall good health, mental balance and the proper functioning of the male reproductive system. (It is also very beneficial for women.)
- Helps to develop memory, energy and courage.
- Recommended for problems of the thyroid and parathyroid glands and metabolism.

8b. Matsyásana
(Fish Posture 2)

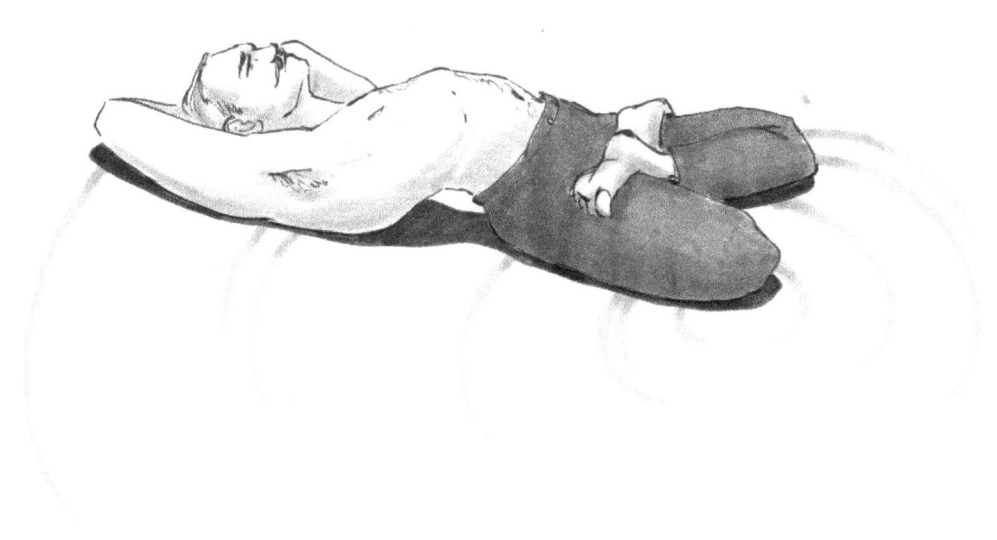

Instructions

1. Place your right foot on your left thigh, and then your left foot on your right thigh, as in *padmásana* (lotus posture). Lie down on your back, keeping your legs in this position.
2. Place your right arm behind your head in such a way that your right hand is touching your left shoulder. Do the same with your left arm, with the left hand touching your right shoulder. Rest you head on your arms.
3. Practise three times, for thirty seconds each time, breathing normally.

- Helps to develop memory, energy and courage.
- Recommended for problems of the thyroid and parathyroid glands and metabolism
- Removes tension in the neck and shoulders.

9. *Naokásana* (Boat Posture)

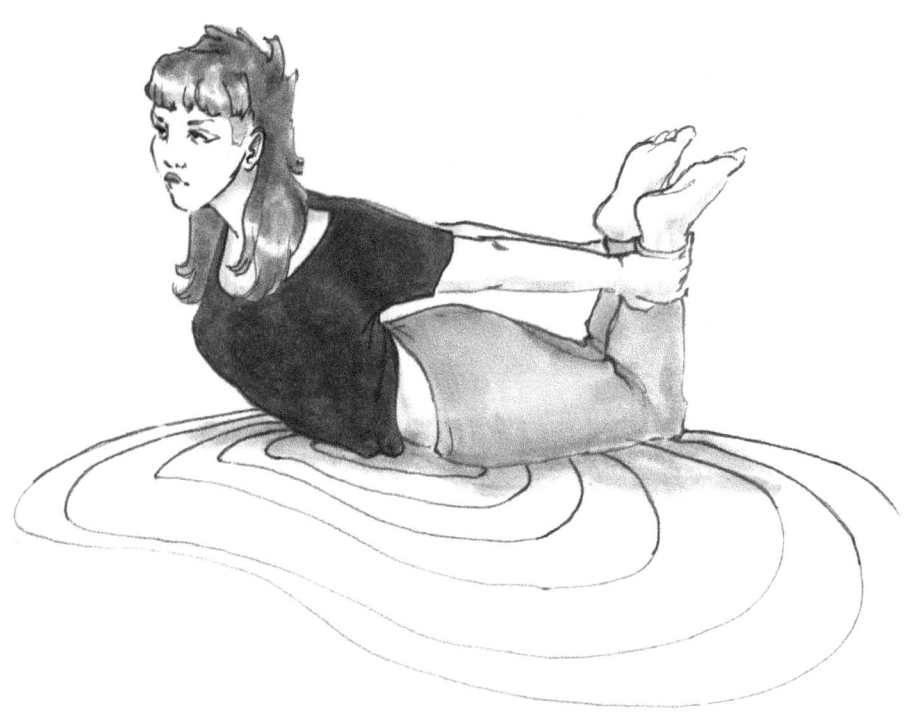

Instructions

1. Lie on your stomach. Bend your knees and hold your ankles with your hands.
2. Breathe in and lift your chest and legs, supporting your weight on your navel. Extend your neck and chest so that your eyes are looking straight ahead.
3. Hold this position for eight seconds, without breathing (breath inhaled). Breathe out and relax your body to the floor. Repeat eight times.

- This is one of the four basic postures recommended for men, to maintain overall good health, mental balance and the proper functioning of the male reproductive system. (It is also very beneficial women).
- Useful for those with weakness in the throat, abdomen and thighs.
- Especially recommended for digestive problems, constipation, etc.
- Helps to maintain the flexibility of the entire body, especially the spine.

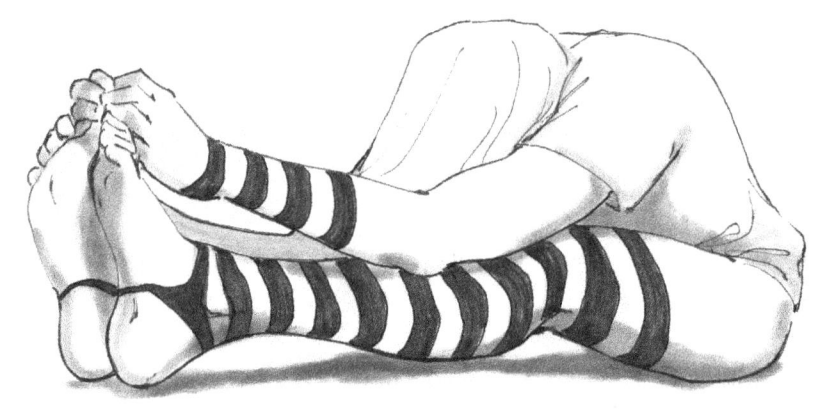

10. *Utkata Paschimottánásana* (Back-Lifting Posture)

Instructions

1. Lie on your back and extend your arms backwards, keeping them close to your ears. Inhale, and then raise your body while exhaling, bending forwards until you face touches your knees, with your arms extended forwards towards your feet. Make sure that your legs remain straight.
2. Grasp both of your big toes with your hands. Hold this position for eight seconds without breathing (breath exhaled).
3. Inhale and return to the original position, lying on the floor with your arms extended backwards. Repeat eight times.

- This is one of the four basic postures recommended for men, to maintain overall good health, mental balance and the proper functioning of the male reproductive system. (It is also very beneficial women.)
- Helpful for those suffering from loss of appetite.
- Helps to relieve stiffness in the spinal cord.
- Tones the stomach muscles.

- *Not recommended for people with liver, spleen or appendix problems, or those suffering from hernia.*

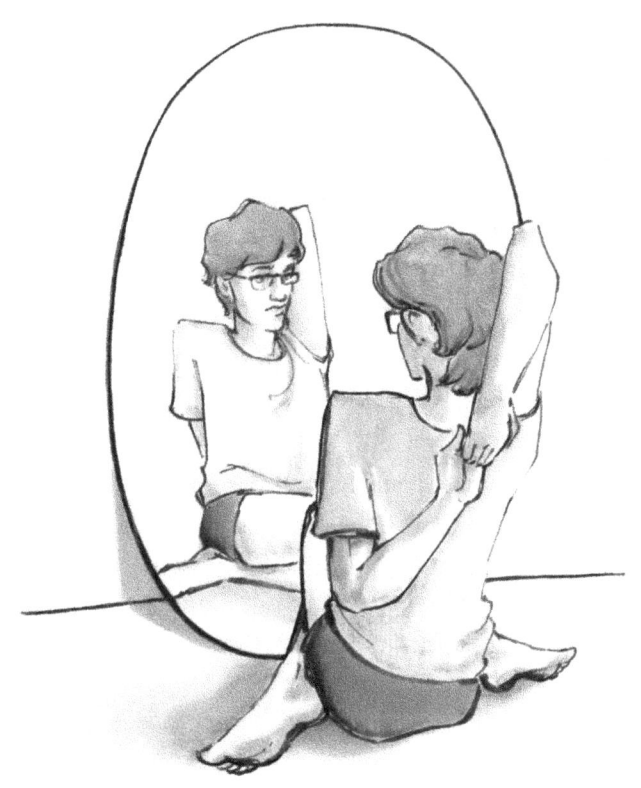

11. *Gomukhásana* (Cow's-Head Posture)

Instructions

1. Sit down on the floor with your legs extended forwards. Place your right leg under your left thigh, so that the right foot is positioned under your left buttocks. Now lift your left leg over your right thigh, so that your left foot is under your right buttocks.
2. Place your left hand on your spine. Then raise your right hand upwards and backwards over your right shoulder, interlocking the fingers of both hands together. Breathing normally, hold this position for thirty seconds.
3. Repeat in the same way but with your arms and legs in the opposite positions. Completing this on both sides is one cycle. Practise four such cycles.

- Beneficial for those suffering from kidney problems, sciatica and piles.
- Useful for maintaining the health and proper functioning of the male reproductive and urinary systems.
- Helps to gain strength and immunity after sickness.

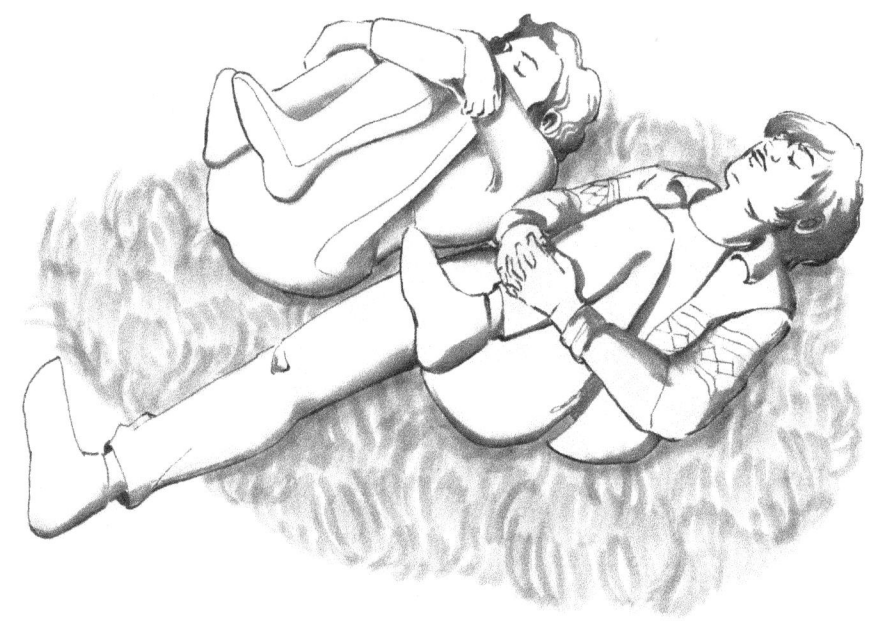

12. *Bhastrikásana* (Bellows Posture)

Instructions

1. Lie on your back, and while breathing out, bend your right leg so that your calf is touching your thigh and your thigh is resting on your chest. Hold your leg firmly with both hands.
2. Hold this position for eight seconds, without breathing (breath exhaled). Breathing in, relax your leg to the floor.
3. Repeat the same with your left leg, and then with both legs together. Repeat this cycle eight times.

- This posture is very effective in alleviating bloating and gas caused by indigestion.
- Beneficial for those suffering from excess fat in the stomach area.
- Recommended for people suffering from high blood pressure.
- Helps alleviate headaches caused by gas, indigestion, or constipation.

13. Mayúrásana
(Peacock Posture)

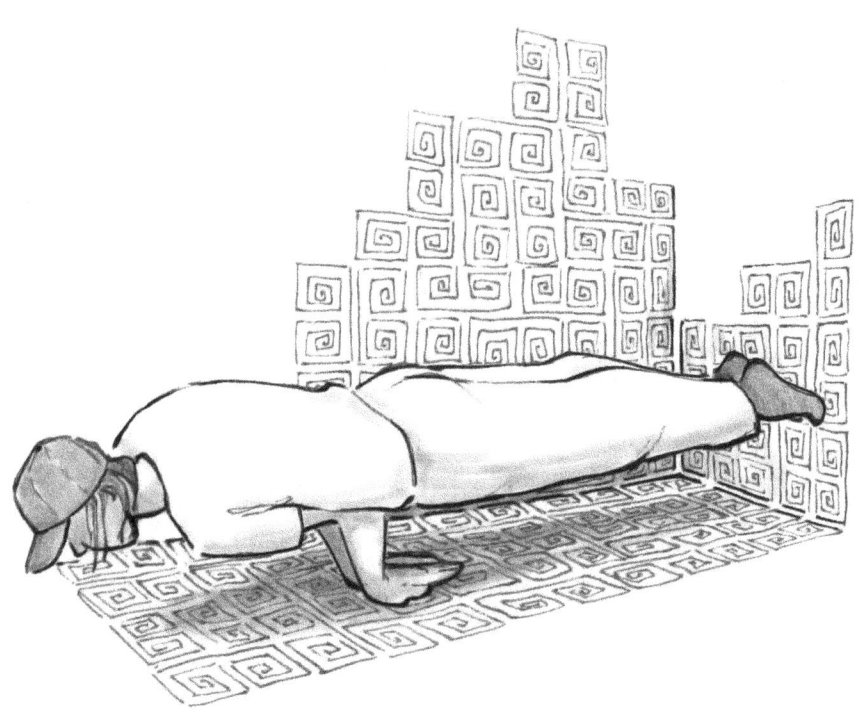

Instructions

1. Sit in a squatting position. Bring your wrists together and then place your palms on the floor, with your fingers pointing towards your feet. Then place your elbows touching your navel and stretch your legs backward.
2. Supporting your weight on your elbows, raise your head and legs from the floor.
3. Hold yourself in this position for thirty seconds, breathing normally. Repeat four times.

- Helps with all kinds of digestive problems, and increases the strength of the digestive system.
- Beneficial for maintaining all-round good health and physical strength.

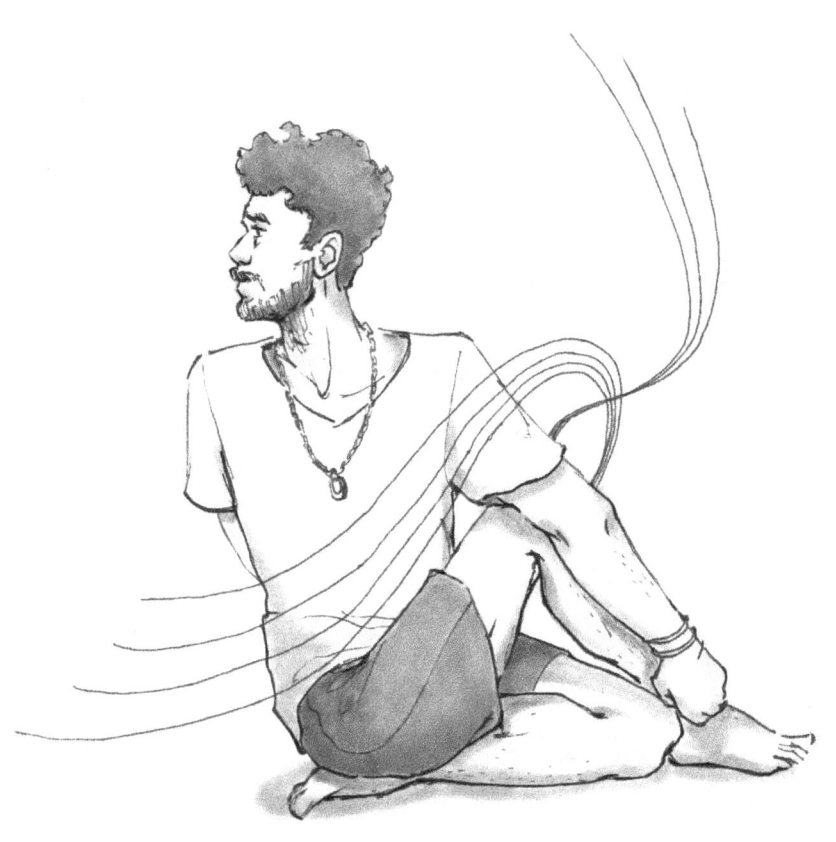

14. *Matsyendrásana*
(Posture of the Yogi Matsyendra)

Instructions

1. Press the perineum with your right heel. Cross your left foot over your right thigh.
2. Hold the big toe of your left foot with your right hand, positioning your right arm along the left side of your left knee.
3. Stretch your left hand backwards across your spine, as if trying to touch your navel with your hand. Turn your neck to the left as far as possible, keeping your eyes focused to the left. Hold this position for thirty seconds, breathing normally.
4. Repeat the same with the positions of the legs and arms reversed. Practise four times on each side, alternating from one side to the other.

- Helps to remove lethargy, tiredness and lack of appetite.
- Beneficial for the lungs.
- Helpful for treating digestive problems.
- Helps to decrease stomach fat.
- Recommended to develop the strength of the knees and neck.
- Helps to strengthen the nerves of the eyes.
- This posture is especially beneficial for men, and helps to maintain the health of the male reproductive and urinary systems. It is not recommended for women except in special circumstances.

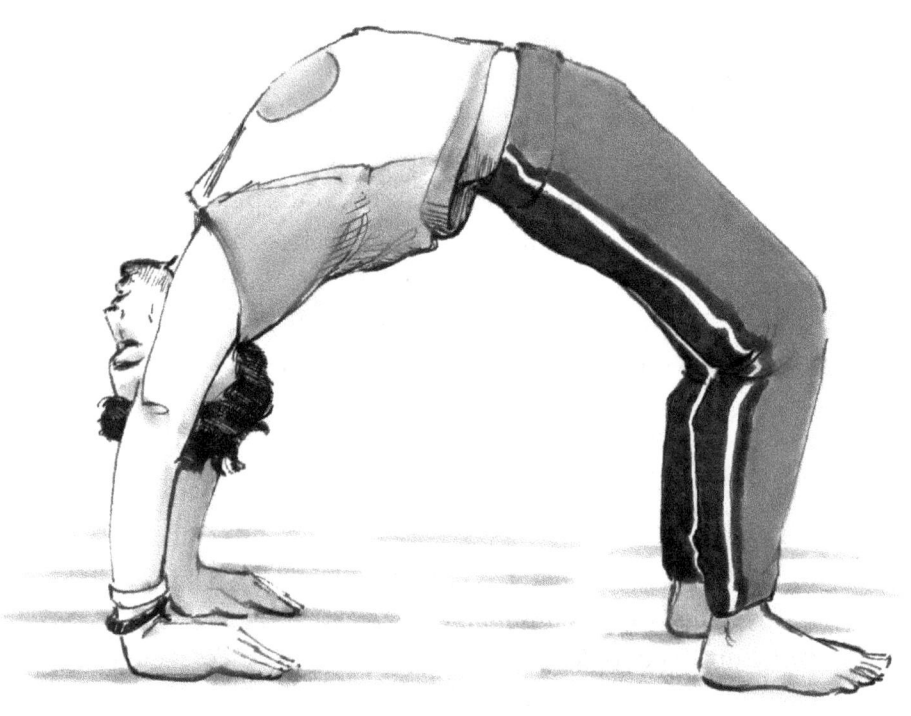

15. *Cakrásana* (Wheel Posture)

Instructions

1. Lie on your back. Bend your legs so as to bring your calves in contact with your thighs. Place your palms on the floor close to your shoulders.
2. Supporting your weight on your feet and palms, raise your head, back and legs until your body takes the form of a wheel or half circle. Inhale when raising the body and exhale as you release yourself from the position. Breathe normally when holding the posture.
3. Hold this position for thirty seconds. Repeat four times.

- Helpful for all kinds of digestive problems, and especially for those who suffer from constipation.
- Helpful for women who suffer from from menstrual pain.
- Helps to maintain the flexibility of the spine and develop strength in the chest, abdomen and thighs.

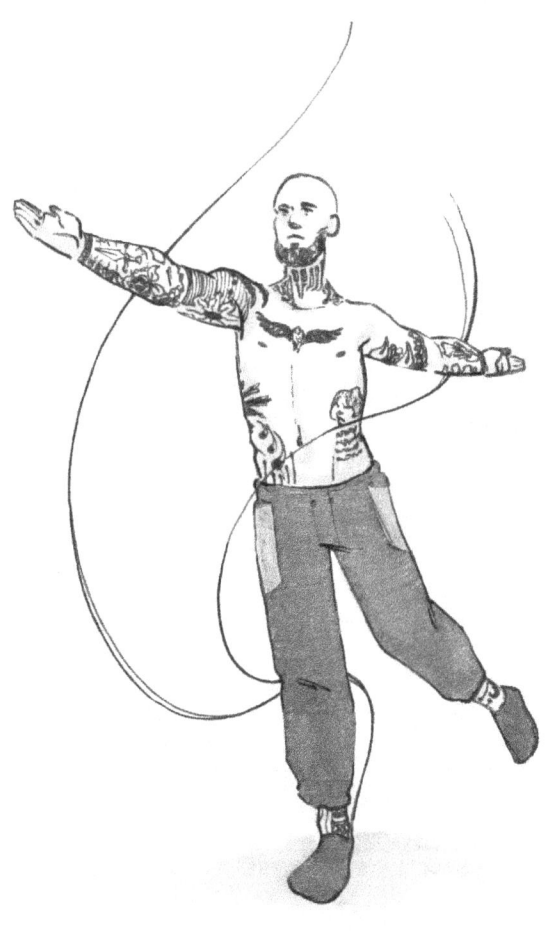

16. *Garudásana* (Eagle Posture)

Instructions

1. Stand straight. Stretch your right leg as far back as possible. Extend your left arm forwards and right arm backwards, keeping both arms parallel to the ground. Your body should remain straight, but the right leg may be bent slightly upwards.
2. Hold this position for thirty seconds, breathing normally.
3. Repeat with the legs and arms in reverse position. This is one cycle. Repeat four cycles.

- Helps to reduce excess weight and to develop physical balance.

17. Tuládańdásana
(Balance Posture)

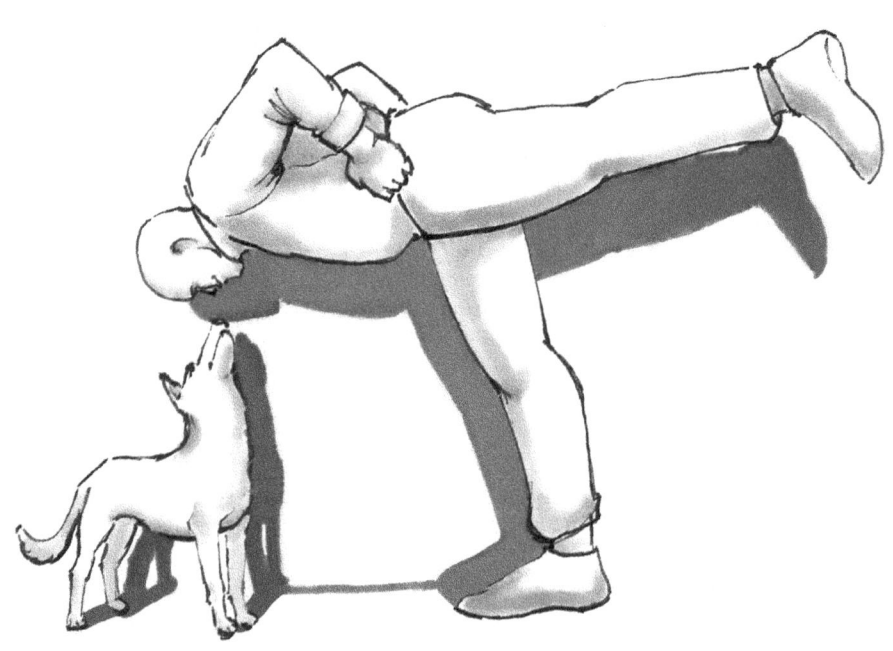

Instructions

1. Standing on your left foot, stretch your right foot backwards, lifting it from the ground. Hold your waist with your hands, then lift your right leg until you entire body is positioned parallel to the floor.
2. Hold this position for thirty seconds, breathing normally.
3. Repeat the same standing on your right foot. This is one cycle. Repeat four cycles.

- Helps to develop strength in the legs.
- Helps to develop balance and coordination.

18. *Sahaja Utkatásana* (Simple Chair Posture)

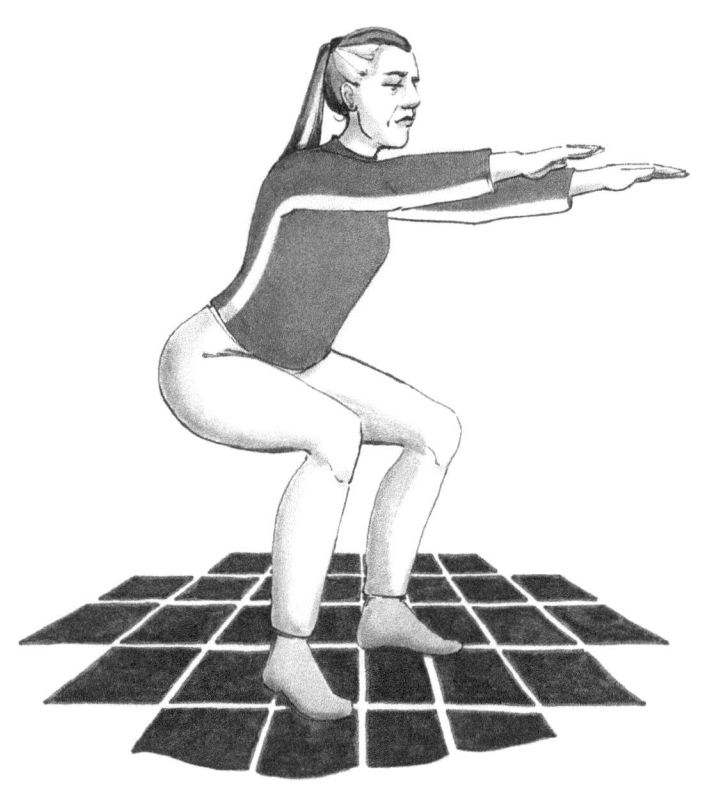

Instructions

1. Seat yourself as if in an imaginary chair. Extend your arms out straight in front of you.
2. Hold this position for thirty seconds, breathing normally. Repeat four times.

- Helps to strengthen the legs and knees.
- Help to alleviate mild sciatica or arthritis in the lower part of the body.

19. Jatila Utkatásana
(Difficult Chair Posture)

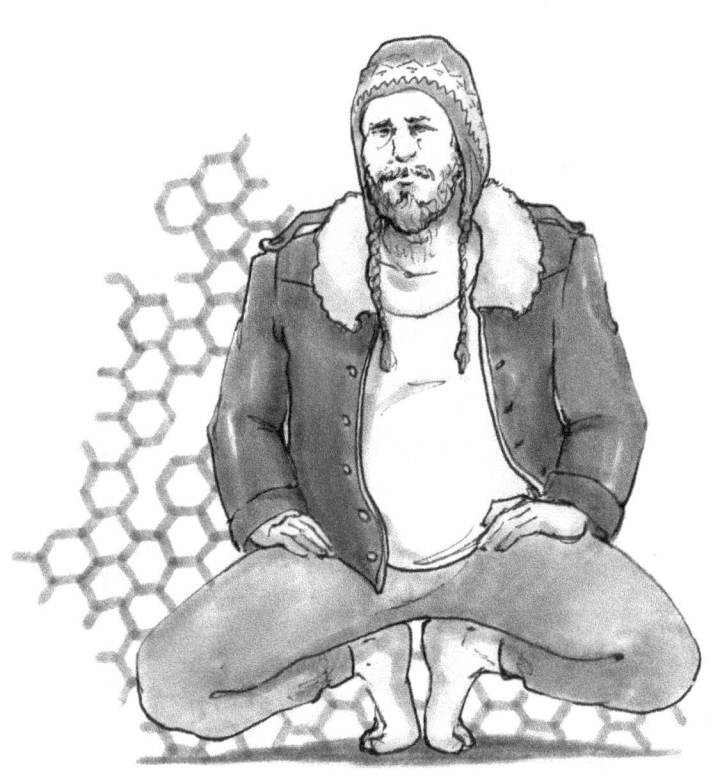

Instructions

1. Sit in a squatting position, with your knees directed outwards, supporting the weight of your body on your toes.
2. Rest your buttocks on your heels and hold your waist with your hands.
3. Hold this position for thirty seconds, breathing normally. Repeat four times.

- Useful for sports-people and those who have to walk for long distances.
- Helps to treat swelling in the legs

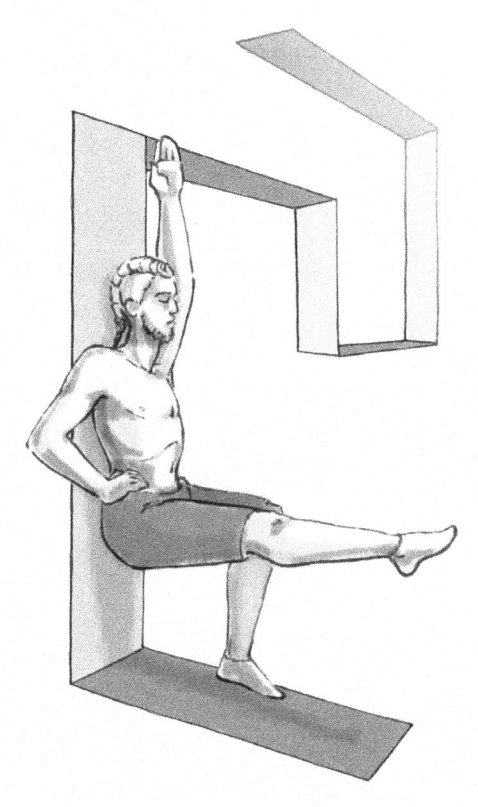

20. Dvisamakońásana
(Double-Right-Angle Posture)

Instructions

1. Bend your knees, taking the position of a chair. Extend your right leg forwards so that it is parallel to the ground, and then raise your left arm upwards. Hold your waist with your right hand. Hold this position for eight seconds, breathing normally.
2. Repeat the same with your left leg stretched forwards. Repeat four times on each side, alternating from one side to the other.

- Increases the strength of the legs and knees.
- Increases balance and coordination.

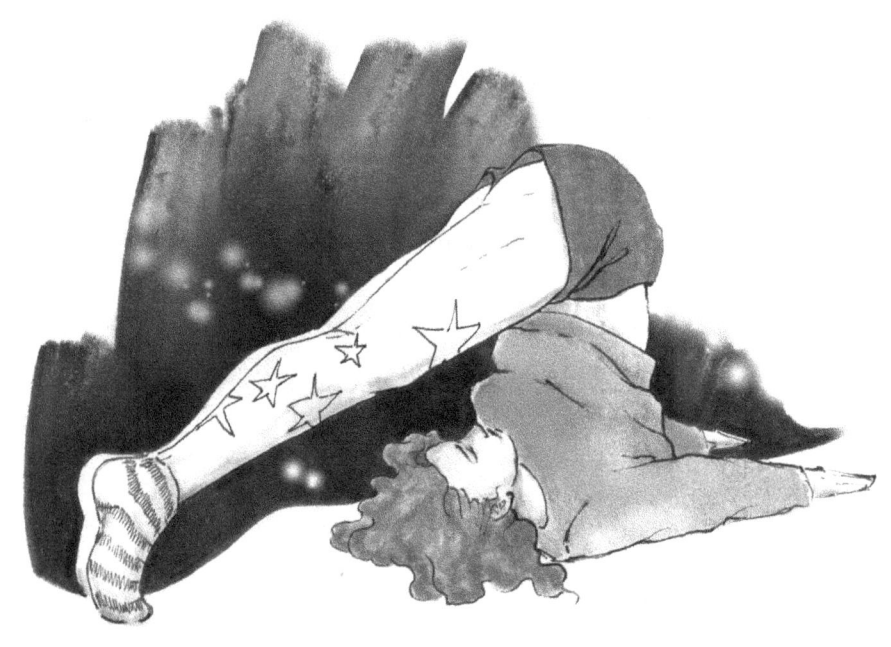

21. *Parvatásana* (Mountain Posture)

Instructions

1. Lie on your back. Raise your body until your weight is resting on your shoulders. Support both sides of your body with your hands.
2. Gradually extend your legs backwards as far as possible until the toes of both feet touch the ground. Release your hands from your back and extend your arms outwards on the floor, palms facing downwards.
3. Hold this position for a maximum of five minutes, breathing normally.
4. As with *sarváungásana* (shoulder-stand), it is recommended to alternate this posture with *matsyamudrá* (fish posture), which should be practised for half the duration of *parvatásana*. For example, do *parvatásana* for three minutes, followed by *matsyamudrá* for one and a half minutes.

- Helpful in treating menstrual problems (menstrual cramps, irregular menstruation, etc.)
- Helpful in treating indigestion.
- Strengthens the shoulders and abdomen.

- *Not recommended for people with heart problems.*

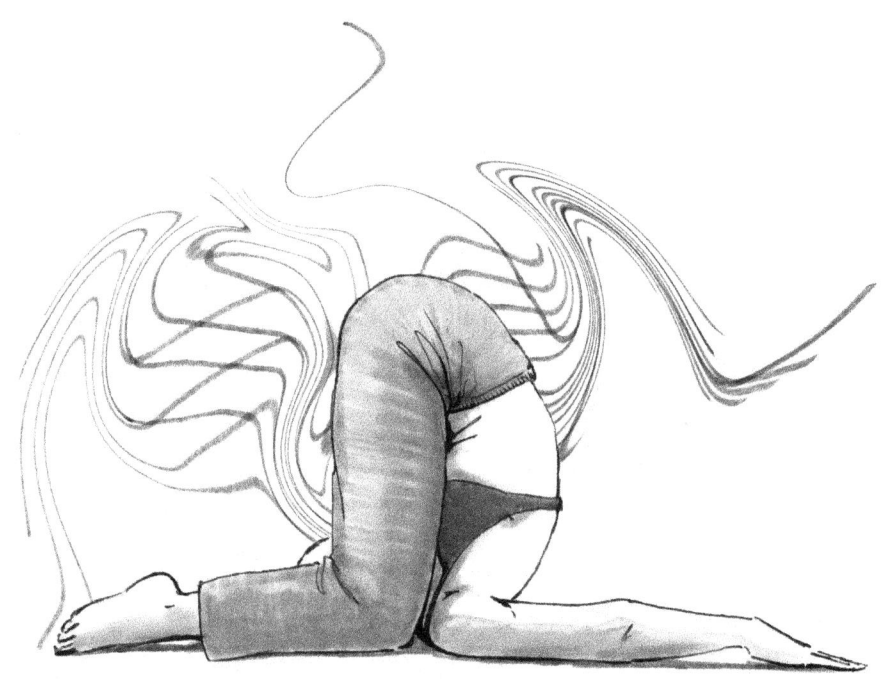

22. *Shivásana* (Posture of Shiva)

Instructions

1. Lie on your back. Raise your body until your weight is resting on your shoulders. Support both sides of your body with your hands.
2. Gradually extend your legs backwards as far as possible until the toes of both feet touch the ground, then lower your knees until they touch the floor, keeping them close to your ears.
3. Release your hands from your back and extend your arms outwards on the floor. Interlock the fingers of both hands firmly together, keeping your hands in contact with the ground.
4. Hold this position for a maximum of five minutes, breathing normally.
5. As with *sarváungásana* (shoulder-stand), it is recommended to alternate this posture with *matsyamudrá* (fish posture), which should be practised for half the duration of *shivásana*. For example, do *shivásana* for three minutes, followed by *matsyamudrá* for one and a half minutes.

- Helpful in treating menstrual problems (menstrual cramps, irregular menstruation).
- Helpful in treating indigestion.
- Strengthens the shoulders, abdomen, neck and waist.

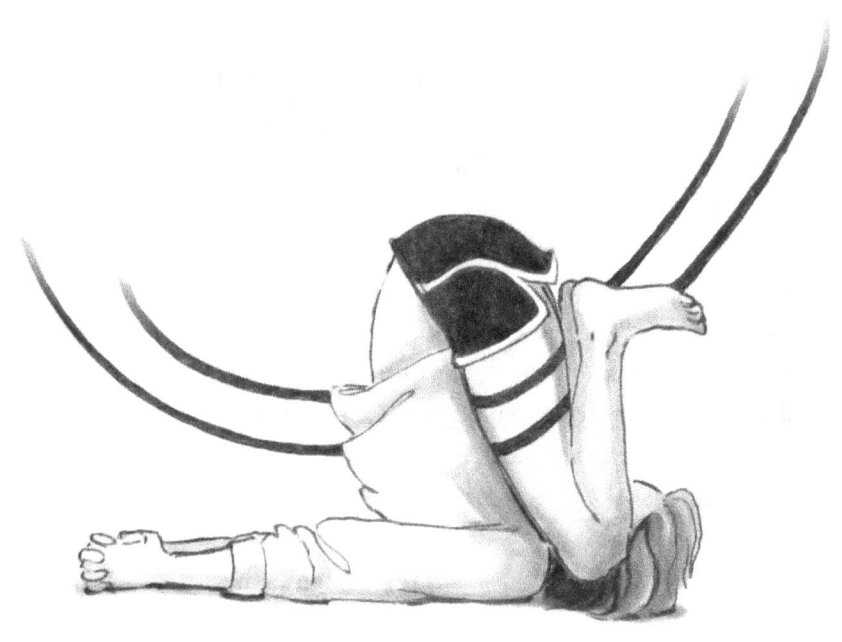

23. *Ardhashivásana*
(Half-Shiva Posture)

Instructions

1. Lie on your back. Raise your body until your weight is resting on your shoulders. Support both sides of your body with your hands.
2. Gradually extend your legs backwards as far as possible until the toes of both feet touch the ground, then lower your knees until they touch the floor, close to your ears.
3. Release your hands from your back and extend your arms outwards on the floor. Interlock your fingers firmly together, keeping your hands in contact with the ground.
4. Raise you feet and calves upwards until your knees are totally bent and your calves are in a vertical position.
5. Hold this position for thirty seconds, breathing normally. Repeat four times.

- Helpful in treating menstrual problems (menstrual cramps, irregular menstruation etc.)
- Helpful in treating indigestion.
- Strengthens the shoulders, abdomen, neck and waist.
- This posture is said to help develop humility.

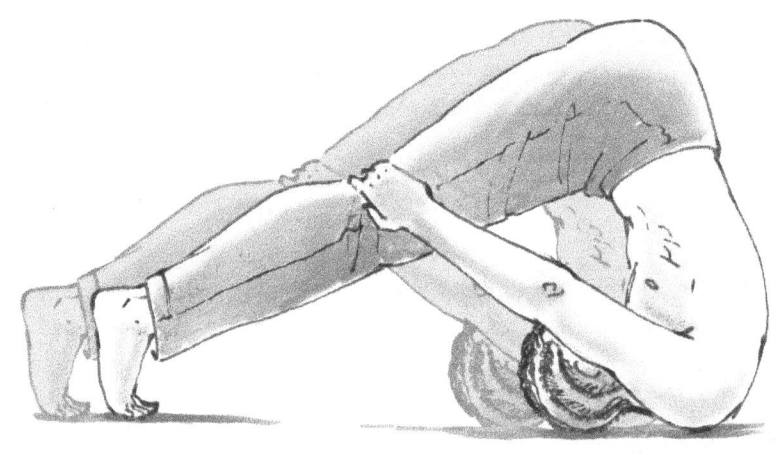

24. *Tejásana* (Energy Posture)

Instructions

1. Lie on your back. Raise your body until your weight is resting on your shoulders. Support both sides of your body with your hands.
2. Gradually extend your legs backwards as far as possible until the toes of both feet touch the ground. Release your hands from your back and extend your arms so that you are holding your legs with your hands.
3. Hold this position for two minutes, breathing normally. Repeat three times.

- This posture helps to increase one's physical energy.
- Helps in obtaining maximum energy from the food that one eats.

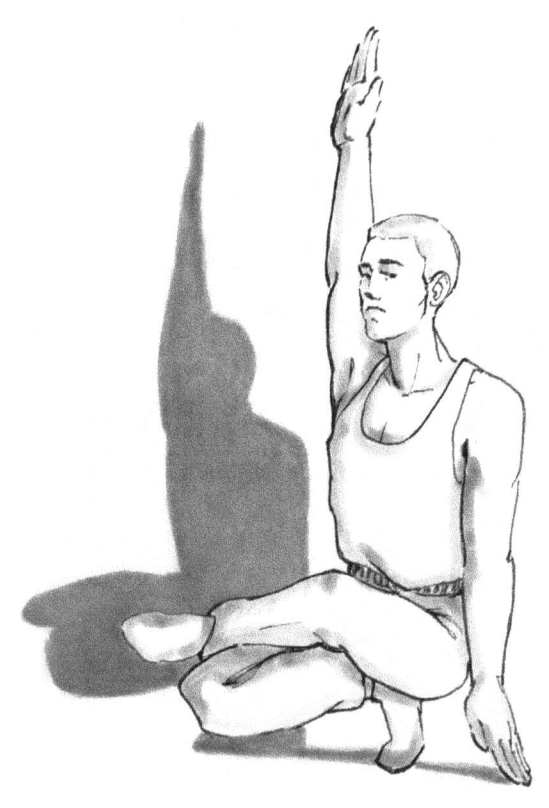

25. *Jiṇānāsana* (Knowledge Posture)

Instructions

1. Sit in a squatting position, with your buttocks resting on your heels, and your hands on the floor a little behind your buttocks and feet.
2. Stretch your left leg forwards a little, and then lift it so as to place your right ankle on the lower part of your left thigh, just above your knee.
3. Raise you left arm to a vertical position, so that it is touching or close to your ear. Keep your eyes looking forwards. Maintain your balance by touching the ground with the fingers of your right hand. Hold this position for thirty seconds, breathing normally.
4. Repeat this process with the legs and arms in the opposite position.
5. Repeat four times on each side, alternating between sides.

- This posture is recommended for developing memory and intelligence, and for those who have difficulty in concentration and study.
- Helps to develop balance and coordination between the left and right sides of the body.

26. *Bhávásana*
(Contemplation Posture)

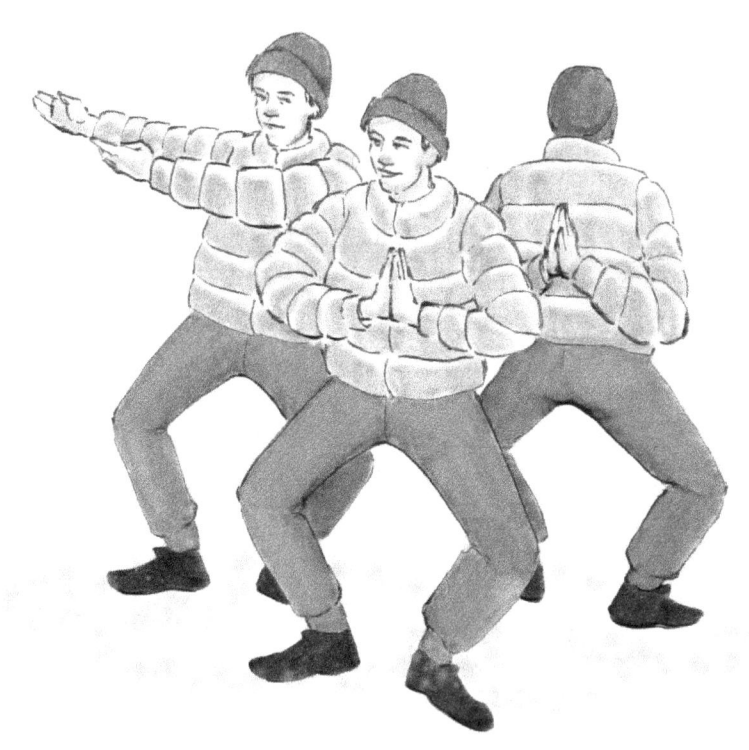

Instructions

1. Stand with your feet apart, at the same distance as your shoulders. Twist your feet so that your toes are facing outwards.
2. Bend your knees and then place your palms together on front of your chest. Imagine that you are focusing on the point between your eyes. Breathing normally, hold this position for eight seconds.
3. Extend both arms to the right, with your left arm touching your chest and stretching to the right as far as possible. Hold this position for eight seconds, breathing normally.
4. Extend your arms to the left in the same way. Hold this position for eight seconds, breathing normally.
5. Place your arms behind your back, with your wrists twisted so that your palms are held together. Hold this position for eight seconds, breathing normally.
6. Repeat this entire sequence four times.

- Helps to develop concentration, memory and a sense of curiosity.
- Helps to remove tension in the shoulders, hips and thighs.
- This a good exercise for the knees and ankles.

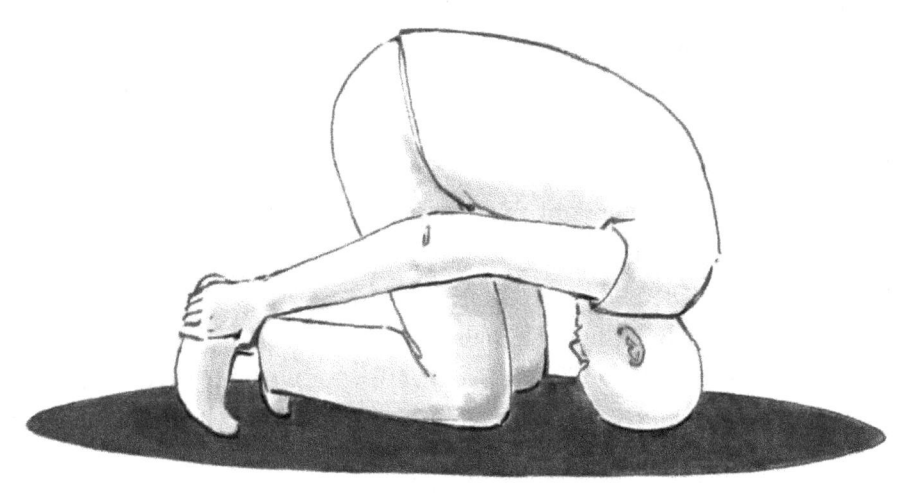

27. Shasháuṇgásana
(Hare Posture)

Instructions

1. Kneel on the floor, with your toes facing inwards (forwards) and your buttocks resting on your heels. Hold your heels with your hands.
2. Breathe out and bend forwards until the top of your head is touching the floor. Your forehead should be close to or touching your knees. Your buttocks may be raised slightly from your heels.
3. Hold this position for eight seconds without breathing (breath exhaled). Repeat eight times.

- Helps to reduce fat in the stomach area.
- Recommended for problems of the thyroid and parathyroid glands.
- Helps to develop a strong memory and improve concentration.
- Helps to develop a calm mind.
- Recommended for people who suffer from insomnia, or who want to meditate but have a lot of difficulty concentrating.

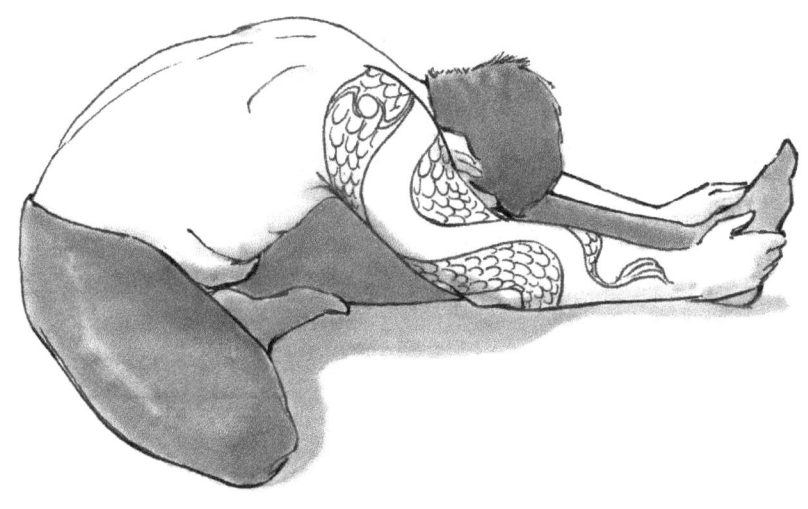

28. Jánushiirásana
(Head-to-Knee Posture)

Instructions

1. Lightly press the perineum with your right heel. Extend your left leg forwards. Exhaling, bend forwards, touching your left knee with your forehead. It is important that your breath is completely exhaled when your forehead reaches your knee.
2. Interlock your fingers around your left foot. Hold this position for eight seconds without breathing (breath exhaled).
3. Release your hands and breathing in, raise your body until you are sitting with your back straight.
4. Change your legs to the opposite position and repeat the same process. This is one cycle. Repeat four cycles.

- Helpful for those suffering from weak digestion or haemorrhoids.
- Recommended for those with a tendency towards melancholy or anxiety.
- Helps to maintain the flexibility of the legs and spine.

29. *Siddhásana*
(Posture of Enlightenment)

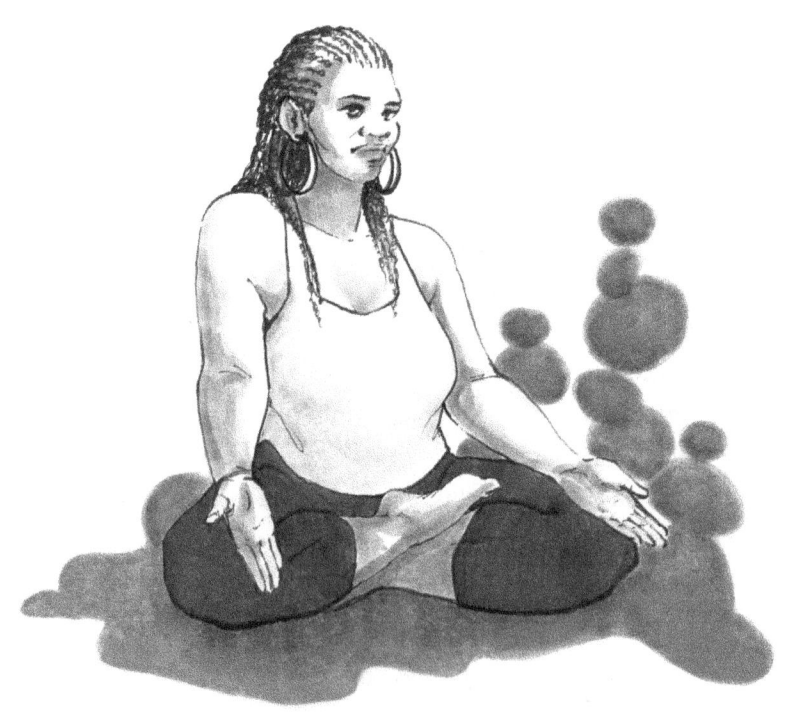

Instructions

1. Press the perineum with your left heel. Then rest your right leg on your left calf, so that your heel is almost pressing the area below the navel. Place your hands, palms facing upwards, on your knees. Maintain this position for as long as you desire, breathing normally.

- This posture is recommended for meditation practice. It helps to maintain the spine in a proper position and aids in concentration.
- Helps to develop patience and calmness of mind.

30. *Padmásana* (Lotus Posture)

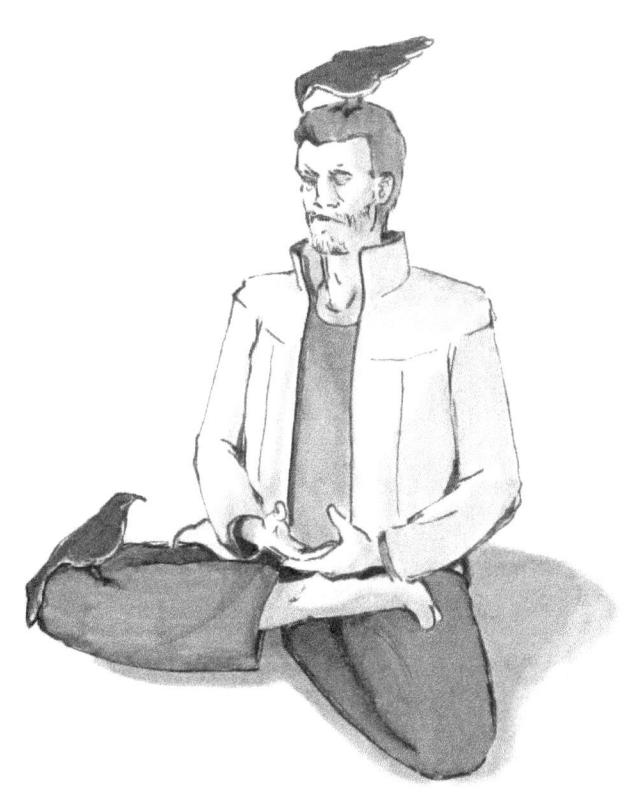

Instructions

1. Place your right foot on your left thigh, and then place your left foot on your right thigh.
2. With your mouth shut, curl your tongue slightly and press it against the roof of your mouth. Place your palms together in your lap, one on top of the other. You can maintain this posture for as long as you like.

- This posture is recommended for meditation practice. It maintains the spine in a proper position and aids in concentration.

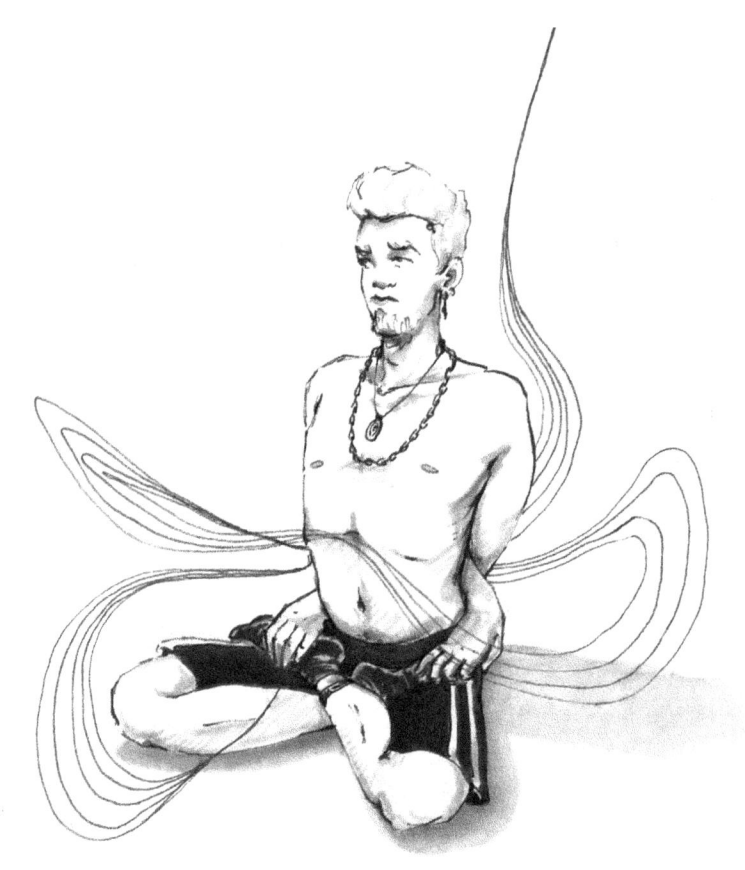

31. Baddha Padmásana (Tied-Lotus Posture)

Instructions

1. Place your right foot on your left thigh, and then place your left foot on your right thigh. Stretch your right hand behind your back until you are grasping your right big toe. Then stretch your left hand behind your back and grasp your left big toe.
2. Hold this position for thirty seconds, breathing normally. Repeat four times.

- Helps develop good posture and flexibility of the spine.
- Removes stiffness in the shoulders.
- Helps to develop concentration and calmness of mind.

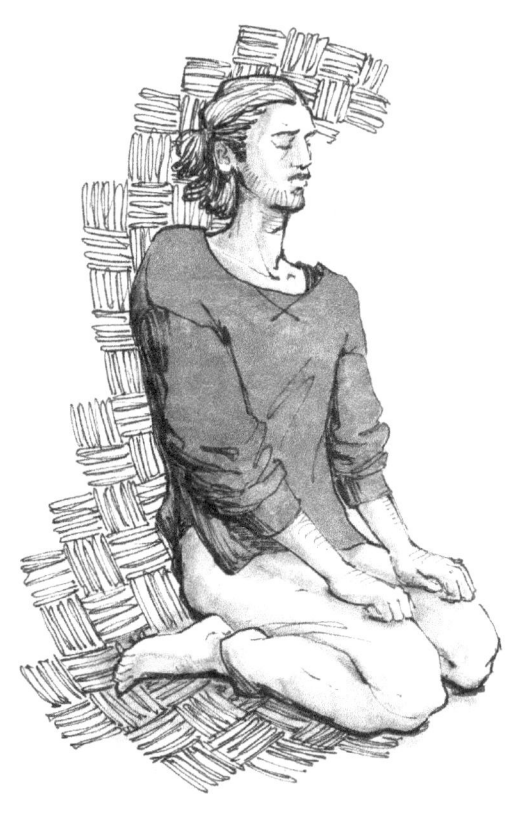

32. *Vajrásana*
(Lightening-Bolt Posture)

Instructions

1. Sit on your knees. Bend your right leg at the knee and then direct your foot outwards so that it is perpendicular to your thigh. Supporting your weight on both hands, direct your left foot outwards in the same way.
2. Now slowly lower your buttocks to the floor. Lift your hands from the floor and place them on your knees.
3. Hold this position for thirty seconds, breathing normally. Repeat four times. In the beginning, practise this posture very carefully.

- Helpful in alleviating sciatica.
- Helpful for those with mild problems in the knee and ankles joints, or in the prevention of knee problems. (If there are serious injuries to the knees, this posture should not be practised.)
- Helps to improve concentration.

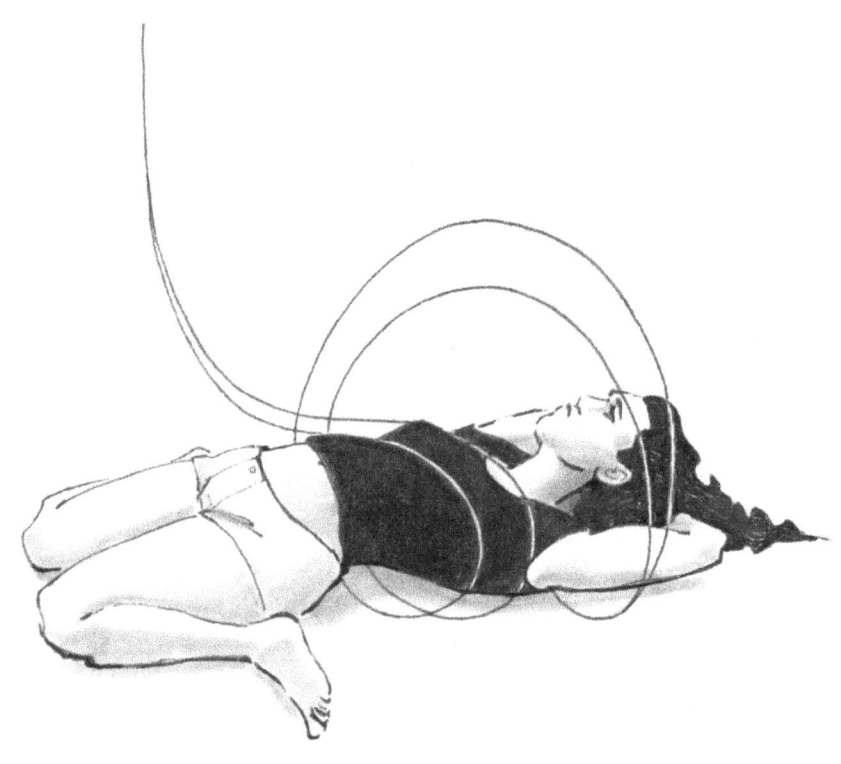

33. Utkata Vajrásana
(Difficult Lightening-Bolt Posture)

Instructions

1. Sit on your knees. Bend your right leg at the knee and then direct your foot outwards so that it is perpendicular to your thigh. Supporting your weight on both hands, direct your left foot outwards in the same way. Now slowly lower your buttocks to the floor. Practice very slowly and carefully in the beginning.
2. Next, lie down slowly, until your back is resting on the floor. Place your hands behind your head.
3. Hold this posture for thirty seconds, breathing normally. Repeat three times.

- Useful for strengthening the knees, abdomen and spinal column.
- Beneficial for people with problems in the knees joints, or to prevent knee problems. (Not to be practised if there is a serious injury to the knees).

34. Shalabhásana
(Locust Posture)

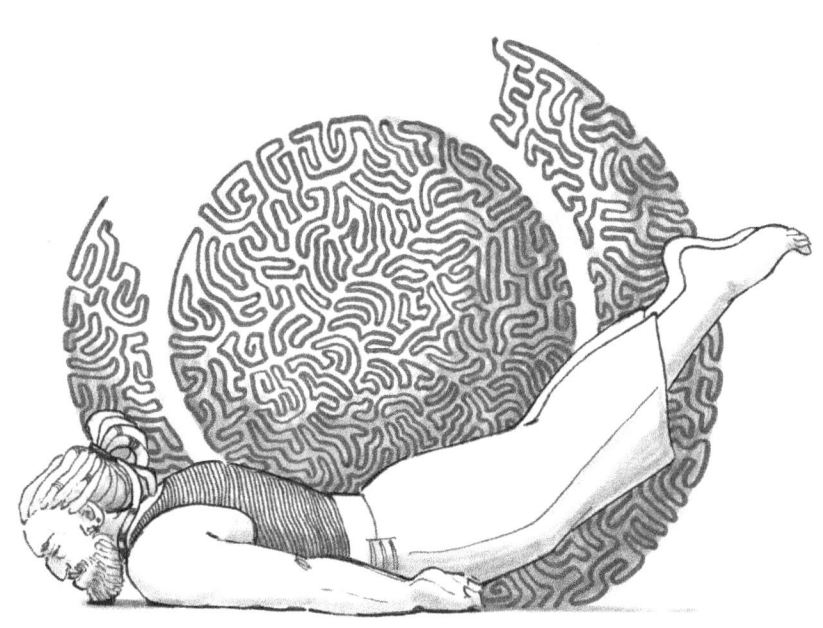

Instructions

1. Lie down on your chest with your hands stretched in the direction of your feet, palms facing upwards. Clenching your fists, raise your legs and waist into the air.
2. Hold this position for thirty seconds, breathing normally. Repeat four times.

- Helps to strengthen the upper half of the body.
- Useful for treating mild pain in the waist area.
- Recommended for those suffering from physical weakness and fatigue.
- Helpful in treating menstrual problems (cramps, excessive bleeding, etc.)

- *This posture should not be practised by those with high blood pressure, or any kind of heart disorder.*

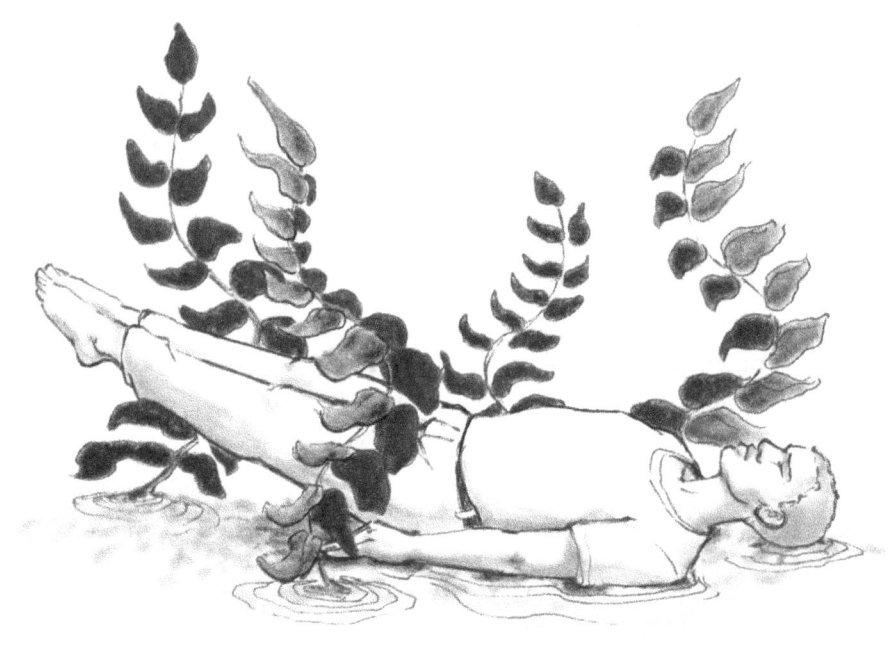

35. *Uśtrásana* (Camel Posture)

Instructions

1. Lie on your back with your arms by your sides.
2. Raise your legs until they are thirty degrees above the floor, without bending your knees.
3. Hold this position for thirty seconds, breathing normally. Repeat four times.

- Helps to strengthen the waist and abdominal region.
- Helps to alleviate sciatica.

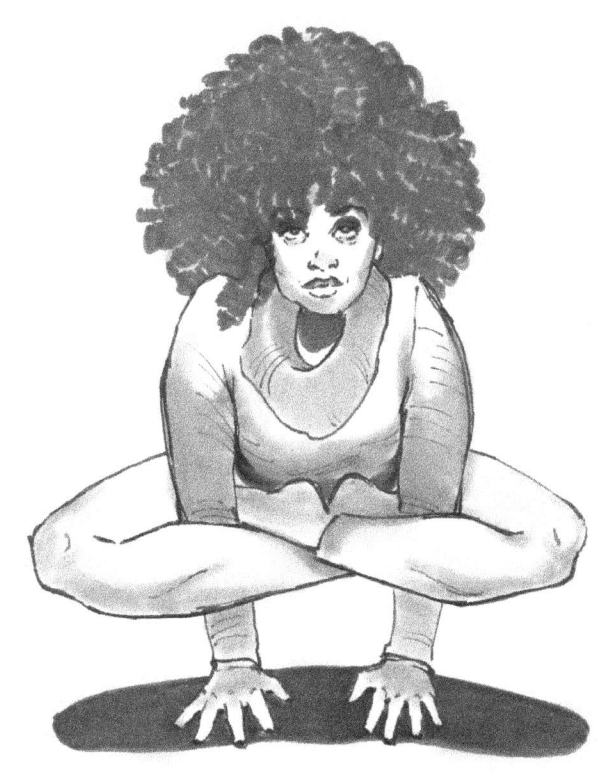

36. *Kukkutásana* (Rooster Posture)

Instructions

1. Place your right foot on your left thigh, and then place your left foot on your right thigh, as in *padmásana* (lotus posture).
2. Insert your arms into the space between your calves and feet, and then lift you body, supporting your weight on your hands. Keep your eyes directed forwards.
3. Hold this position for thirty seconds, breathing normally. Repeat four times.

- Helps to strengthen the arms and wrists.
- Strengthens the digestive system.

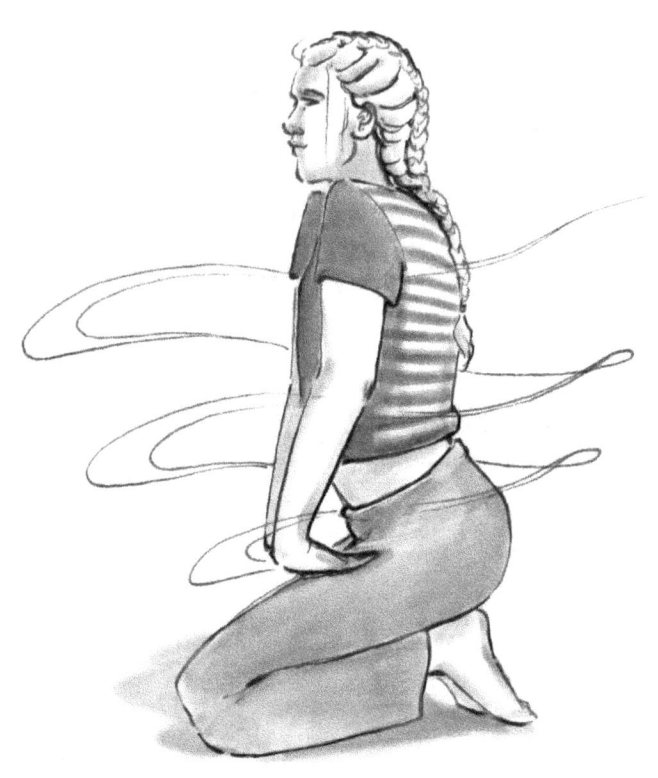

37. Viirásana (Hero's Posture)

Instructions

1. Sit on your knees. Place your feet in an almost vertical position, with your toes facing backwards, pointing away from your body. Lower your buttocks so that it is resting on your feet. Your weight will rest on your toes.
2. Place your hands on your thighs, with your fingers pointing inwards. Try to maintain your spine erect. Concentrate your eyes on the tip of your nose. Hold this position for as long as you like, breathing normally.

- This posture is recommend to develop courage and concentration.
- Strengthens the nerves of the eyes.
- Stretches the muscles of the toes, feet and ankles.

38. *Kúrmakásana* (Tortoise Posture)

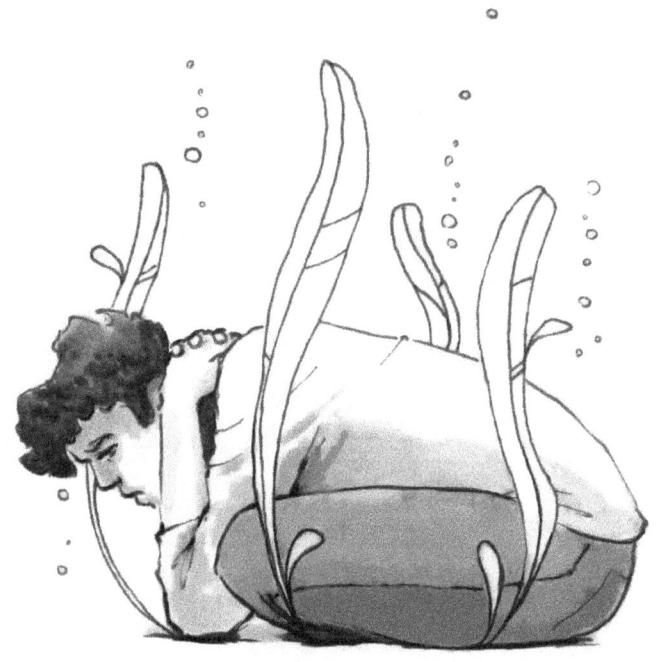

Instructions

1. Place your right foot on your left thigh, and then place your left foot on your right thigh, as in *padmásana* (lotus posture).
2. Insert your arms into the spaces between your calves and feet, so that your elbows touch the floor. Bend your back forwards and place your hands behind your neck, with your fingers interlinked.
3. Stretch your neck slightly so that your face and eyes are directed forwards.
4. Hold this position for thirty seconds, breathing normally. Repeat four times.

- Helps to maintain the flexibility of the entire body.
- Removes tension in the neck and spine.
- Helps to develop patience.

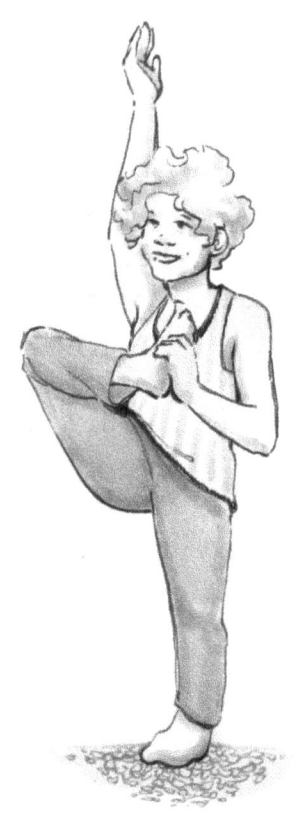

39. *Granthimuktásana* (Knot-Loosening Posture)

Instructions

1. Standing on your feet, hold your left ankle with your right hand. Stretch your leg and foot in such a way that your big toe is directed towards your nose. You should try to touch your right nostril with your toe.
2. Raise your left arm to a vertical position. Hold this position for eight seconds, breathing normally.
3. Repeat the same with the other leg. Practice four times on each side, alternating from one side to the other.

- Removes stiffness of the muscles and joints in the hips, thighs, knees and ankles.
- Helps to develop balance and coordination.

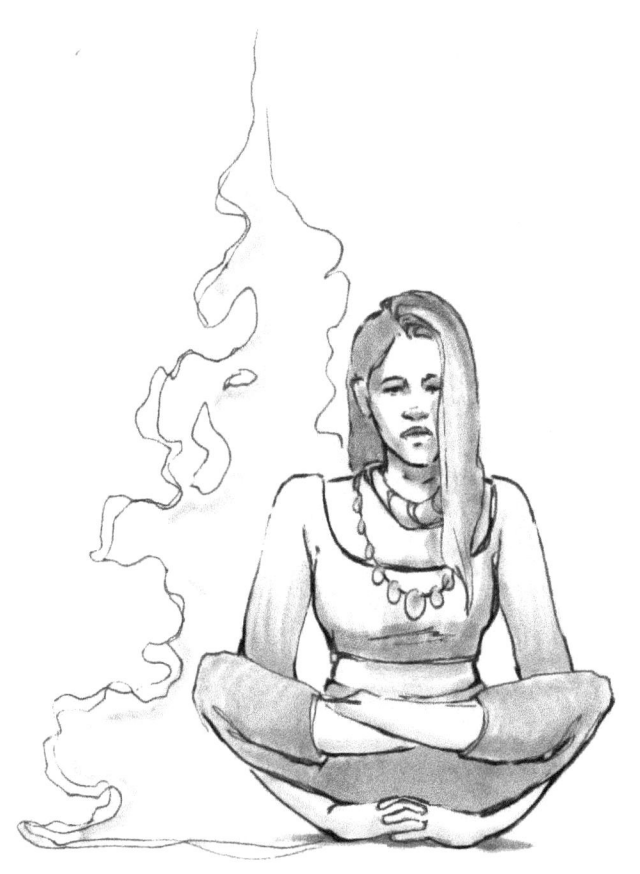

40. *Maṅdukásana* (Frog Posture)

Instructions

1. Place your right foot on your left thigh, and then your left foot on your right thigh, as in *padmásana* (lotus posture).
2. Raise your legs so that your weight is resting on your buttocks. Wrap your arms around your legs, behind your knees, in such a way that your hands meet below your thighs. Interlock your fingers with your palms facing towards the floor.
3. Using your hands and wrists, lift your buttocks and entire body over your hands, as if jumping forwards. Repeat this movement three times.
4. Repeat the same, but starting with your hands behind your buttocks, and jumping backwards three times.
5. Repeat this series of movements (jumping forwards and then backwards three times each) three times.

- Helps to strengthen the arms and wrists.
- Good for developing balance and coordination.
- Helps to control the appetite.

41. Utkata Kúrmakásana
(Difficult Tortoise Posture)

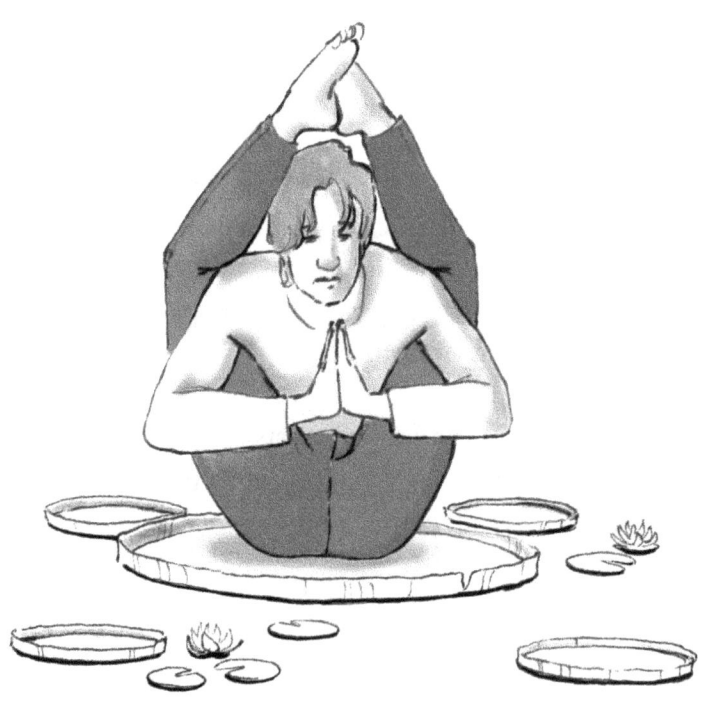

Instructions

1. Stretch your right leg behind your right shoulder, placing your foot behind your neck. Then stretch your left leg behind your left shoulder, so that your left ankle is touching your right ankle.
2. Place your palms together in front of your chest.
3. Hold this position for thirty seconds, breathing normally. Repeat four times.

- Stretches all the joints and muscles. This posture is considered to contain the benefits of all the other yoga postures combined.
- Good for concentration and coordination.

42. *Shavásana*
(Relaxation Posture)

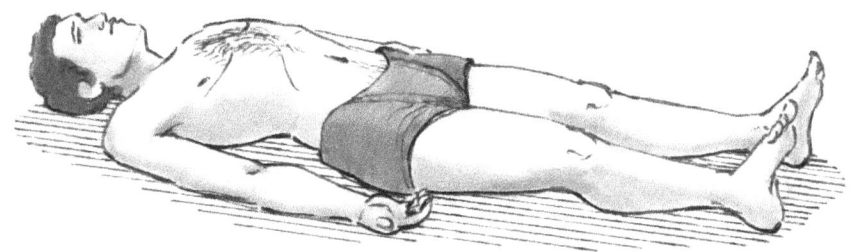

Instructions

1. Lie on your back with your eyes closed. Your legs should be slightly apart with your feet in a relaxed position. Your arms should be placed slightly away from your body, palms facing upwards.
2. Lie like this for two to ten minutes, breathing slowly and deeply.

- This posture should be practised at the end of any yoga routine, after completing the other postures and self-massage. It can also be practised between postures. It helps the muscles, nerves and glands to assimilate the benefits of the postures.
- Helps to enter into a state of deep relaxation.
- Helps to relax the muscles of the eyes and face.
- Useful for those who suffer from anxiety, restlessness and high-blood pressure.
- This posture is especially recommended for those who have to do intellectual work for long periods of time. In this case, it is recommended to practise it for up to ten minutes.

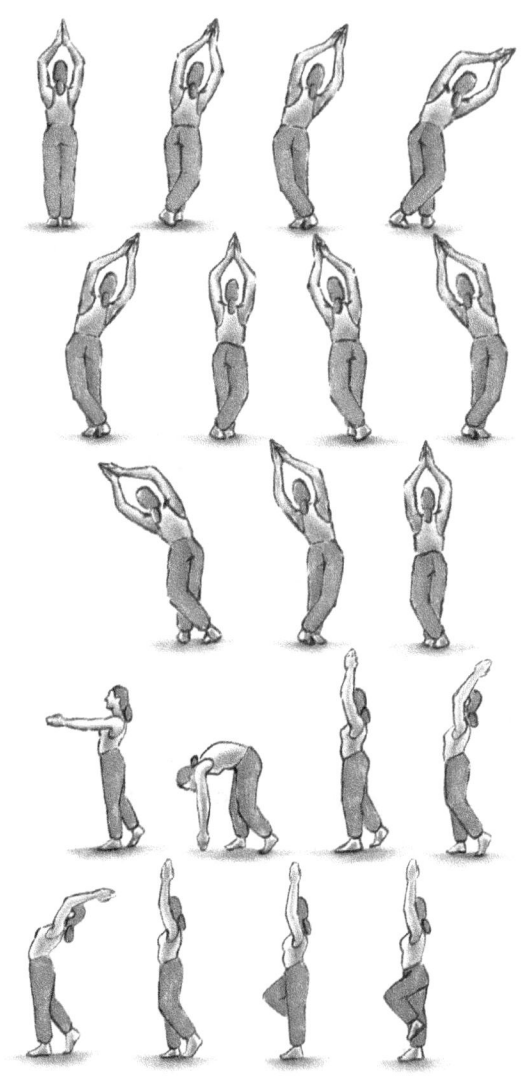

Kaoshikii

Kaoshikii is a yogic dance designed to maintain the flexibility of the entire body. The movements are made in such a way as to prevent and alleviate stiffness, joint pain and arthritis and to energise and create a feeling of lightness in the body. Aside from good flexibility, Kaoshikii has many other benefits: it stimulates the flow of lymph throughout the body; balances the nervous and endocrine systems; and aids good digestion and a properly functioning metabolism. It is highly recommended for the maintenance of healthy reproductive and urinary systems, especially for women who suffer from menstrual pain or irregular menstruation.

As well as its physical benefits, Kaoshikii is said to have various psychological benefits when practised regularly. Through its energising and balancing effect on the glands and nerves, it helps to develop good concentration and strength of mind, and to overcome lethargy, low self-esteem, fear complexes, self-doubt, etc. The name 'Kaoshikii' means 'a dance to open up the layers of the mind.'

When performing Kaoshikii, there is a synchronisation of the arms and legs: for one movement of the legs, there is a parallel movement of the arms. First, the arms are stretched upwards, palms together. You should try to keep them straight and positioned close to your ears. To begin, bend your right knee and place your right foot behind your left heel, touching the floor with your big toe. At the same time, complete the first movement of the arms as indicated in the diagram. Continue with all the movements as indicated. At the end, you will stamp each foot on the ground lightly, one after the other, with the arms remaining straight upwards. You can then continue the whole cycle again from the beginning without pausing between cycles, repeating as many times as you like. Kaoshikii can be practised at any time, though it is best incorporated into a yoga routine, before or after completing the yoga postures or after the relaxation session, as your prefer. It can also be practised during pregnancy if desired, when adjusted to the physical condition of the expecting mother.

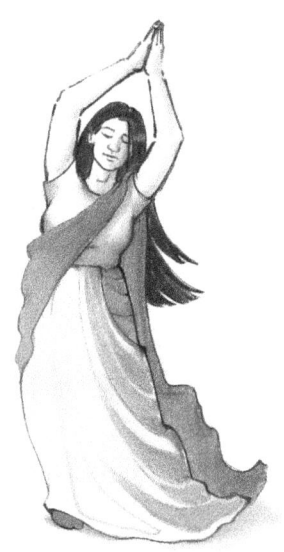

Model of an Effective Yoga Routine:

1. Time of Day:

The best time of day to practice yoga asanas is in the morning before breakfast or in the evening before eating dinner. It is not recommended to do asanas on a full-stomach or for around two hours after eating a meal.

2. Freshen Up!

Before doing Yoga, you should be fresh, clean and relaxed. If you have taken a bath or shower beforehand, that's perfect. Otherwise, your can do a 'half-bath', a quick and easy yogic technique to freshen up the body and senses.

- First, if needed, use the toilet, and then rinse the urinary organ with cool water. This leaves the body fresh and clean. It is actually a common habit in many parts of the world.
- If the weather is very hot, you can wet the navel with a little water. This is one of the hottest areas of the body, and cooling it helps to cool down the whole body.
- Pour cool water from your knees to your feet and elbows to hands.
- Breathing in, place a handful of water in your mouth. Holding your breath whilst keeping the water in your mouth, splash water into your open eyes at least twelve times. After this, spit out the water.
- Wash your face and neck.

3. Yoga Postures (Asanas)

Select three to six yoga asanas. Start with the simpler postures, and then lead up to the more difficult ones. If you don't know which postures to start with, you can try the three basic postures for women, or four basic postures for men.

4. Self-Massage
It is highly recommended to do a quick self-massage after completing your asana routine. This is massage of the skin, so you do not need to use pressure or to apply any kind of oil.

To start, place your hands over your closed eyes and relax the muscles of your eyes and face. Then pass your hands over your head, face, ears and neck. Proceed to your shoulders, arms, and entire body until your legs and feet, lightly but firmly rubbing the skin, giving special focus to the joints. You can apply a bit of extra pressure to the soles of your feet.

5. Relaxation
A yoga routine should always be finished with a few minutes of relaxation. Lie on your back in the relaxation posture, breathing deeply. Remain like this for two to ten minutes.

6. Kaoshikii
You can incorporate this yogic dance into your asana routine. You can do it at the beginning, after completing the postures, or after the relaxation, according to personal preference.

7. A Short Pause
If possible, it is best not to drink or eat immediately after practising asanas. Try to wait at least a short time, around fifteen minutes. If you can fit it into your routine, it is also beneficial to take a short walk in the fresh air.

The Sattvic Diet

According to Yoga and Ayurveda, there is a close link between the food we eat and our physical and psychological state. Food is divided into three categories according to their influence upon the glands and mind. These categories are: *'sattvic'* (sentient); *'rajasic'* (mutative); and *'tamasic'* (static). To get the maximum benefit from a regular yoga routine, especially if you also wish to combine it with a meditation practice, it recommended to follow a *sattvic* diet, with small quantities of *rajasic* foods if desired. Although this may seem like too much of a challenge, many yoga and meditation practitioners report that with regular practise they naturally start to preference these foods, and the change comes much more easily than expected.

'Sattvic' food includes almost all vegetarian foods, with a few exceptions. Most vegetables, fruits, grains and pulses, herbs and spices, as well as dairy products are *sattvic*.

'Rajasic' foods include coffee, tea, chocolate, and other caffeinated drinks. In very cold climates these foods are considered to become *sattvic*.

'Tamasic' foods include meat products (red and white meat and fish), alcohol and intoxicating drugs, garlic, onion and mushroom. Although garlic and onion have some medicinal qualities, their overall effect on the mind when consumed regularly is considered to be negative. One of the most obvious benefits of leaving out these foods from your diet it that the odour of the body and breath almost instantly improve. Although many of the foods in this category are very common and it may seem difficult to avoid them, the best way is to try it out and see how you feel over time.

Other Publications of Interest:

Yama Niyama: Yogic Ethics for a Balanced Mind
A Tapasiddha
ISBN: 978-0473487546

An in-depth analysis of the concept of ethics within the yogic world-view and as a part of spiritual meditation, this book discusses the principles of Yama Niyama from the perspective of psychology and philosophy in modern language suitable to the western student. Yama Niyama are considered as the base upon which empathy, trust, self-reflection and a coherent personality can develop, thus facilitating the practice of meditation and introspection. One becomes aware of the subconscious source of one's emotional patterns and the effect that these have on one's self-esteem and social interactions. In addition to an understanding of yogic ethics, the reader will also gain insights into many other aspects of the philosophy and psychology of Tantra Yoga.

Recognising the relativity of our daily experiences yet based in certain essential archetypical truths, Yama Niyama serve to produce an integrated personality on the individual level and the foundations of a healthy society collectively. Yama Niyama work to challenge one's individual limitations and preconceptions, producing a continuous process of mental expansion and deepening awareness of what is means to be human.

Intangible Things Set Free
A Tapasiddha
ISBN: 978-0473498047

This unexpected and touching collection of poetry roams between the vulnerability of sadness and joy expressing themselves through a love that searches continuously for its own essence. The author's words come from an uncommon place of simplicity and honesty that touches on something universal yet at once completely personal. As the title suggests, these are poems to set free that which is intangible, misunderstood or too often denied within us and within humanity, as the varied and so often apparently opposing aspects of our psyche seek for meaning and harmony.

The poems offer a rare insight insight into the often misunderstood path of the author's tantra yoga practice, whilst at the same time, perhaps surprisingly and in an uncommon act of perception and balance, are free from any unnatural imposition from it.

www.ingramcontent.com/pod-product-compliance
Lightning Source LLC
Chambersburg PA
CBHW080400030426
42334CB00024B/2946